P9-CBW-895

IN DEFENSE OF FOOD

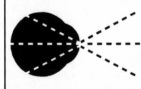

This Large Print Book carries the
Seal of Approval of N.A.V.H.

In Defense of Food

AN EATER'S MANIFESTO

Michael Pollan

THORNDIKE PRESS
A part of Gale, Cengage Learning

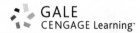

Detroit • New York • San Francisco • New Haven, Conn • Waterville, Maine • London

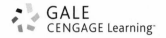

GALE
CENGAGE Learning™

A portion of this book first appeared in *The New York Times Magazine* under the title "Unhappy Meals."
Thorndike Press, a part of Gale, Cengage Learning.

Thorndike Press® Large Print Nonfiction.
The text of this Large Print edition is unabridged.
Other aspects of the book may vary from the original edition.
Set in 16 pt. Plantin.
Printed on permanent paper.

LIBRARY OF CONGRESS CATALOGING-IN-PUBLICATION DATA

Pollan, Michael.
   In defense of food : an eater's manifesto / by Michael Pollan.
     p. cm.
   "The text of this Large Print edition is unabridged."
   Includes bibliographical references.
   ISBN-13: 978-1-4104-0537-1 (hardcover : alk. paper)
   ISBN-10: 1-4104-0537-0 (hardcover : alk. paper)
   1. Nutrition. 2. Food habits. 3. Large type books. I. Title.
RA784.P643 2008a
613.2—dc22   2007050670

Published in 2008 by arrangement with The Penguin Press, a member of Penguin Group (USA) Inc.

Printed in the United States of America
1 2 3 4 5 6 7 12 11 10 09 08

For Ann and Gerry,
*With gratitude for your loyal friendship
and inspired editing*

CONTENTS

INTRODUCTION:
AN EATER'S MANIFESTO

Eat food. Not too much. Mostly plants.

That, more or less, is the short answer to the supposedly incredibly complicated and confusing question of what we humans should eat in order to be maximally healthy.

I hate to give the game away right here at the beginning of a whole book devoted to the subject, and I'm tempted to complicate matters in the interest of keeping things going for a couple hundred more pages or so. I'll try to resist, but will go ahead and add a few more details to flesh out the recommendations. Like, eating a little meat isn't going to kill you, though it might be better approached as a side dish than as a main. And you're better off eating whole fresh foods rather than processed food products. That's what I mean by the recommendation to "eat food," which is not quite as simple as it sounds. For while it used to be that food was all you *could* eat, today there are

9

thousands of other edible foodlike substances in the supermarket. These novel products of food science often come in packages elaborately festooned with health claims, which brings me to another, somewhat counterintuitive, piece of advice: If you're concerned about your health, you should probably avoid products that make health claims. Why? Because a health claim on a food product is a strong indication it's not really food, and food is what you want to eat.

You can see how quickly things can get complicated.

I started on this quest to identify a few simple rules about eating after publishing *The Omnivore's Dilemma* in 2006. Questions of personal health did not take center stage in that book, which was more concerned with the ecological and ethical dimensions of our eating choices. (Though I've found that, in most but not all cases, the best ethical and environmental choices also happen to be the best choices for our health — very good news indeed.) But many readers wanted to know, after they'd spent a few hundred pages following me following the food chains that feed us, "Okay, but what should I *eat*? And now that you've been to the feedlots, the food-processing plants, the organic factory farms, and the local farms and ranches, what do *you* eat?"

Fair questions, though it does seem to me a symptom of our present confusion about food that people would feel the need to consult a journalist, or for that matter a nutritionist or doctor or government food pyramid, on so basic a question about the conduct of our everyday lives as humans. I mean, what other animal needs professional help in deciding what it should eat? True, as omnivores — creatures that can eat just about anything nature has to offer and that in fact need to eat a wide variety of different things in order to be healthy — the "What to eat" question is somewhat more complicated for us than it is for, say, cows. Yet for most of human history, humans have navigated the question without expert advice. To guide us we had, instead, Culture, which, at least when it comes to food, is really just a fancy word for your mother. What to eat, how much of it to eat, what order in which to eat it, with what and when and with whom have for most of human history been a set of questions long settled and passed down from parents to children without a lot of controversy or fuss.

But over the last several decades, mom lost much of her authority over the dinner menu, ceding it to scientists and food marketers (often an unhealthy alliance of the two) and, to a lesser extent, to the government, with its ever-shifting dietary guidelines, food-labeling rules, and perplexing pyramids. Think about it: Most of us no longer eat what our mothers ate as children or, for that matter, what our mothers fed us as children. This is, historically speaking, an unusual state of affairs.

My own mother grew up in the 1930s and 1940s eating a lot of traditional Jewish-American fare, typical of families who recently emigrated from Russia or Eastern Europe: stuffed cabbage, organ meats, cheese blintzes, kreplach, knishes stuffed with potato or chicken liver, and vegetables that often were cooked in rendered chicken or duck fat. I never ate any of that stuff as a kid, except when I visited my grandparents. My mother, an excellent and adventurous cook whose own menus were shaped by the cosmopolitan food trends of New York in the 1960s (her influences would have included the 1964 World's Fair; Julia Child and Craig Claiborne; Manhattan restaurant menus of the time; and of course the rising drumbeat of food marketing) served us a rotating menu that each week completed a culinary world tour: beouf bourguignon or beef Stroganoff on Monday; coq au vin or oven-fried chicken (in a Kellogg's Corn-flakes crust) on Tuesday; meat loaf or Chinese pepper steak on Wednesday (yes, there was a *lot* of beef); spaghetti pomodoro with Italian sausages on Thursday; and on her weekend nights off, a Swanson's TV dinner or Chinese takeout. She cooked with Crisco or Wesson oil rather than chicken or duck fat and used margarine rather than butter because she'd absorbed the nutritional orthodoxy of the time, which held that these more up-to-date fats were better for our health. (Oops.)

Nowadays I don't eat any of that stuff — and neither does my mother, who has moved on too. Her parents wouldn't recognize the foods we put on the table, except maybe the butter, which is back. Today in America the culture of food is changing *more* than once a generation, which is historically unprecedented — and dizzying.

What is driving such relentless change in the American diet? One force is a thirty-two-billion-dollar food-marketing machine that thrives on change for its own sake. Another is the constantly shifting ground of nutrition science that, depending on your point of view, is steadily advancing the frontiers of our knowledge about diet and health or is just changing its mind a lot because it is a flawed science that knows much less than it cares to admit. Part of what drove my grandparents' food culture from the American table was official scientific opinion, which, beginning in the 1960s, decided that animal fat was a deadly substance. And then there were the food manufacturers, which stood to make very little money from my grandmother's cooking, because she was doing so much of it from scratch — up to and including rendering her own cooking fats. Amplifying the "latest science," they managed to sell her daughter on the virtues of hydrogenated vegetable oils, the ones that we're now learning may be, well, deadly substances.

Sooner or later, everything solid we've been told about the links between our diet and our health seems to get blown away in the gust of the most recent study. Consider the latest findings. In 2006 came news that a low-fat diet, long believed to protect against cancer, may do no such thing — this from the massive, federally funded Women's Health Initiative, which has also failed to find a link between a low-fat diet and the risk of coronary heart disease. Indeed, the whole nutritional orthodoxy around dietary fat appears to be crumbling, as we will see.

In 2005 we learned that dietary fiber might not, as we'd been confidently told for years, help prevent colorectal cancers and heart disease. And then, in the fall of 2006, two prestigious studies on omega-3 fats published at the same time came to strikingly different conclusions. While the Institute of Medicine at the National Academy of Sciences found little conclusive evidence that eating fish would do your heart much good (and might hurt your brain, because so much fish is contaminated with mercury), a Harvard study brought the hopeful piece of news that simply by eating a couple of servings of fish each week (or by downing enough fish oil tablets) you could cut your risk of dying from a heart attack by more than a third. It's no wonder that omega-3 fatty acids are poised to become the oat bran of our time as food scientists rush to microencapsulate fish and algae oil and blast it into such formerly all-terrestrial foods as bread and pasta, milk and yogurt and cheese, all of which will soon, you can be sure, spout fishy new health claims. (I hope you remember the relevant rule.)

By now you're probably feeling the cognitive dissonance of the supermarket shopper or science-section reader as well as some nostalgia for the simplicity and solidity of the first few words of this book. Words I'm still prepared to defend against the shifting winds of nutritional science and food-industry marketing, and will. But before I do, it's important to understand how we arrived at our present state of nutritional confusion and anxiety. That is the subject of the first portion of this book, "The Age of Nutritionism."

The story of how the most basic questions about what to eat ever got so complicated reveals a great deal about the institutional imperatives of the food industry, nutrition science, and — ahem — journalism, three parties that stand to gain much from wide-spread confusion surrounding the most elemental question an omnivore confronts. But humans deciding what to eat without professional guidance — something they have been doing with notable success since coming down out of the trees — is seriously unprofitable if you're a food company, a definite career loser if you're a nutritionist, and just plain boring if you're a newspaper editor or reporter. (Or, for that matter, an eater. Who wants to hear, yet again, that you should "eat more fruits and vegetables"?) And so like a large gray cloud, a great Conspiracy of Scientific Complexity has gathered around the simplest questions of nutrition — much to the advantage of everyone involved. Except perhaps the supposed beneficiary of all this nutritional advice: us, and our health and happiness as eaters. For the most important thing to know about the campaign to professionalize dietary advice is that it has not made us any healthier. To the contrary: As I argue in part one, most of the nutritional advice we've received over the last half century (and in particular the advice to replace the fats in our diets with carbohydrates) has actually made us less healthy and considerably fatter.

My aim in this book is to help us reclaim our health and happiness as eaters. To do this requires an exercise that might at first blush seem unnecessary, if not absurd: to offer a defense of food and the eating thereof. That food and eating stand in need of a defense might seem counterintuitive at a time when "overnutrition" is emerging as a more serious threat to public health than undernutrition. But I contend that most of what we're consuming today is no longer, strictly speaking, food at all, and how we're consuming it — in the car, in front of the TV, and, increasingly, alone — is not really eating, at least not in the sense that civilization has long understood the term. Jean-

Anthelme Brillat-Savarin, the eighteenth-century gastronomist, drew a useful distinction between the alimentary activity of animals, which "feed," and humans, who eat, or dine, a practice, he suggested, that owes as much to culture as it does to biology.

But if food and eating stand in need of a defense, from whom, or what, do they need defending? From nutrition science on one side and from the food industry on the other — and from the needless complications around eating that together they have fostered. As eaters we find ourselves increasingly in the grip of a Nutritional Industrial Complex — comprised of well-meaning, if error-prone, scientists and food marketers only too eager to exploit every shift in the nutritional consensus. Together, and with some crucial help from the government, they have constructed an ideology of nutritionism that, among other things, has convinced us of three pernicious myths: that what matters most is not the food but the "nutrient"; that because nutrients are invisible and incomprehensible to everyone but scientists, we need expert help in deciding what to eat; and that the purpose of eating is to promote a narrow concept of physical health. Because food in this view is foremost

18

a matter of biology, it follows that we must try to eat "scientifically" — by the nutrient and the number and under the guidance of experts.

If such an approach to food doesn't strike you as the least bit strange, that is probably because nutritionist thinking has become so pervasive as to be invisible. We forget that, historically, people have eaten for a great many reasons other than biological necessity. Food is also about pleasure, about community, about family and spirituality, about our relationship to the natural world, and about expressing our identity. As long as humans have been taking meals together, eating has been as much about culture as it has been about biology.

That eating should be foremost about bodily health is a relatively new and, I think, destructive idea — destructive not just of the pleasure of eating, which would be bad enough, but paradoxically of our health as well. Indeed, no people on earth worry more about the health consequences of their food choices than we Americans do — and no people suffer from as many diet-related health problems. We are becoming a nation of orthorexics: people with an unhealthy obsession with healthy eating.*

The scientists haven't tested the hypothesis yet, but I'm willing to bet that when they do they'll find an inverse correlation between the amount of time people spend worrying about nutrition and their overall health and happiness. This is, after all, the implicit lesson of the French paradox, so-called not by the French (*Quel paradoxe?*) but by American nutritionists, who can't fathom how a people who enjoy their food as much as the French do, and blithely eat so many nutrients deemed toxic by nutritionists, could have substantially lower rates of heart disease than we do on our elaborately engineered low-fat diets. Maybe it's time we confronted the American paradox: a notably unhealthy population preoccupied with nutrition and diet and the idea of eating healthily.

I don't mean to suggest that all would be

Orthorexia — from the Greek "ortho-" (right and correct) + "exia" (appetite) = right appetite. The term was first proposed in 1996 by the American physician Steven Bratman. Though orthorexia is not yet an eating disorder recognized by the *Diagnostic and Statistical Manual of Mental Disorders,* academic investigation is under way.

well if we could just stop worrying about food or the state of our dietary health: *Let them eat Twinkies!* There are in fact some very good reasons to worry. The rise of nutritionism reflects legitimate concerns that the American diet, which is well on its way to becoming the world's diet, has changed in ways that are making us increasingly sick and fat. Four of the top ten causes of death today are chronic diseases with well-established links to diet: coronary heart disease, diabetes, stroke, and cancer. Yes, the rise to prominence of these chronic diseases is partly due to the fact that we're not dying earlier in life of infectious diseases, but only partly: Even after adjusting for age, many of the so-called diseases of civilization were far less common a century ago — and they remain rare in places where people don't eat the way we do.

I'm speaking, of course, of the elephant in the room whenever we discuss diet and health: "the Western diet." This is the subject of the second part of the book, in which I follow the story of the most radical change to the way humans eat since the discovery of agriculture. All of our uncertainties about nutrition should not obscure the plain fact that the chronic diseases that now kill most of us can be traced directly to the industrialization of our food: the rise of highly processed foods and refined grains; the use of chemicals to raise plants and animals in huge monocultures; the super-abundance of cheap calories of sugar and fat produced by modern agriculture; and the narrowing of the biological diversity of the human diet to a tiny handful of staple crops, notably wheat, corn, and soy. These changes have given us the Western diet that we take for granted: lots of processed foods and meat, lots of added fat and sugar, lots of *every*thing — except vegetables, fruits, and whole grains.

That such a diet makes people sick and fat we have known for a long time. Early in the twentieth century, an intrepid group of doctors and medical workers stationed overseas observed that wherever in the world people gave up their traditional way of eating and adopted the Western diet, there soon followed a predictable series of Western diseases, including obesity, diabetes, cardiovascular diseases, and cancer. They called these the Western diseases and, though the precise causal mechanisms were (and remain) uncertain, these observers had little doubt these chronic diseases shared a common etiology: the Western diet.

What's more, the traditional diets that the

new Western foods displaced were strikingly diverse: Various populations thrived on diets that were what we'd call high fat, low fat, or high carb; all meat or all plant; indeed, there have been traditional diets based on just about any kind of whole food you can imagine. What this suggests is that the human animal is well adapted to a great many different diets. The Western diet, however, is not one of them.

Here, then, is a simple but crucial fact about diet and health, yet, curiously, it is a fact that nutritionism cannot see, probably because it developed in tandem with the industrialization of our food and so takes it for granted. Nutritionism prefers to tinker with the Western diet, adjusting the various nutrients (lowering the fat, boosting the protein) and fortifying processed foods rather than questioning their value in the first place. Nutritionism is, in a sense, the official ideology of the Western diet and so cannot be expected to raise radical or searching questions about it.

But we can. By gaining a firmer grasp on the nature of the Western diet — trying to understand it not only physiologically but also historically and ecologically — we can begin to develop a different way of thinking about food that might point a path out of our predicament. In doing so we have two sturdy — and strikingly hopeful — facts to guide us: first, that humans historically have been healthy eating a great many different diets; and second, that, as we'll see, most of the damage to our food and health caused by the industrialization of our eating can be reversed. Put simply, we can escape the Western diet and its consequences.

This is the burden of the third and last section of *In Defense of Food:* to propose a couple dozen personal rules of eating that are conducive not only to better health but also to greater pleasure in eating, two goals that turn out to be mutually reinforcing.

These recommendations are a little different from the dietary guidelines you're probably accustomed to. They are not, for example, narrowly prescriptive. I'm not interested in telling you what to have for dinner. No, these suggestions are more like eating algorithms, mental devices for thinking through our food choices. Because there is no single answer to the question of what to eat, these guidelines will produce as many different menus as there are people using them.

These rules of thumb are also not framed in the vocabulary of nutrition science. This is not because nutrition science has nothing important to teach us — it does, at least when it avoids the pitfalls of reductionism and overconfidence — but because I believe we have as much, if not more, to learn about eating from history and culture and tradition. We are accustomed in all matters having to do with health to assuming science should have the last word, but in the case of eating, other sources of knowledge and ways of knowing can be just as powerful, sometimes more so. And while I inevitably rely on science (even reductionist science) in attempting to understand many questions about food and health, one of my aims in this book is to show the limitations of a strictly scientific understanding of something as richly complex and multifaceted as food. Science has much of value to teach us about food, and perhaps someday scientists will "solve" the problem of diet, creating the nutritionally optimal meal in a pill, but for now and the foreseeable future, letting the scientists decide the menu would be a mistake. They simply do not know enough.

You may well, and rightly, wonder who am I to tell you how to eat? Here I am advising you to reject the advice of science and industry — and then blithely go on to offer my own advice. So on whose authority do I purport to speak? I speak mainly on the authority of tradition and common sense. Most of what we need to know about how to eat we already know, or once did until we allowed the nutrition experts and the advertisers to shake our confidence in common sense, tradition, the testimony of our senses, and the wisdom of our mothers and grandmothers.

Not that we had much choice in the matter. By the 1960s or so it had become all but impossible to sustain traditional ways of eating in the face of the industrialization of our food. If you wanted to eat produce grown without synthetic chemicals or meat raised on pasture without pharmaceuticals, you were out of luck. The supermarket had become the only place to buy food, and real food was rapidly disappearing from its shelves, to be replaced by the modern cornucopia of highly processed foodlike products. And because so many of these novelties deliberately lied to our senses with fake sweeteners and flavorings, we could no longer rely on taste or smell to know what we were eating.

Most of my suggestions come down to strategies for escaping the Western diet, but before the resurgence of farmers' markets, the rise of the organic movement, and the renaissance of local agriculture now under way across the country, stepping outside the conventional food system simply was not a realistic option for most people. Now it is. We are entering a postindustrial era of food; for the first time in a generation it is possible to leave behind the Western diet without having also to leave behind civilization. And the more eaters who vote with their forks for a different kind of food, the more commonplace and accessible such food will become. Among other things, this book is an eater's manifesto, an invitation to join the movement that is renovating our food system in the name of health — health in the very broadest sense of that word.

I doubt the last third of this book could have been written forty years ago, if only because there would have been no way to eat the way I propose without going back to the land and growing all your own food. It would have been the manifesto of a crackpot. There was really only one kind of food on the national menu, and that was whatever industry and nutritionism happened to be serving. Not anymore. Eaters have real choices now, and those choices have real consequences, for our health and the health of the land and the health of our food culture — all of which, as we will see, are inextricably linked. That anyone should need to write a book advising people to "eat food" could be taken as a measure of our alienation and confusion. Or we can choose to see it in a more positive light and count ourselves fortunate indeed that there is once again real food for us to eat.

■ ■ ■ ■

I
THE AGE OF
NUTRITIONISM

■ ■ ■ ■

ONE:
FROM FOODS TO
NUTRIENTS

If you spent any time at all in a supermarket in the 1980s, you might have noticed something peculiar going on. The food was gradually disappearing from the shelves. Not literally vanishing — I'm not talking about Soviet-style shortages. No, the shelves and refrigerated cases still groaned with packages and boxes and bags of various edibles, more of them landing every year in fact, but a great many of the traditional supermarket foods were steadily being replaced by "nutrients," which are not the same thing. Where once the familiar names of recognizable comestibles — things like eggs or breakfast cereals or snack foods — claimed pride of place on the brightly colored packages crowding the aisles, now new, scientific-sounding terms like "cholesterol" and "fiber" and "saturated fat" began rising to large-type prominence. More important than mere foods, the presence or absence of these invisible substances was now generally believed to confer health benefits on their eaters. The implicit message was that foods, by comparison, were coarse, old-fashioned, and decidedly unscientific things — who could say *what* was in them really? But nutrients — those chemical compounds and minerals in foods that scientists have identified as important to our health — gleamed with the promise of scientific certainty. Eat more of the right ones, fewer of the wrong, and you would live longer, avoid chronic diseases, and lose weight.

Nutrients themselves had been around as a concept and a set of words since early in the nineteenth century. That was when William Prout, an English doctor and chemist, identified the three principal constituents of food — protein, fat, and carbohydrates — that would come to be known as macronutrients. Building on Prout's discovery, Justus von Liebig, the great German scientist credited as one of the founders of organic chemistry, added a couple of minerals to the big three and declared that the mystery of animal nutrition — how food turns into flesh and energy — had been solved. This is the very same Liebig who identified the macronutrients in soil — nitrogen, phosphorus, and potassium (known to farmers and gardeners by their periodic table initials, N, P, and K). Liebig claimed that all that plants need to live and grow are these three chemicals, period. As with the plant, so with the person: In 1842, Liebig proposed a theory of metabolism that explained life strictly in terms of a small handful of chemical nutrients, without recourse to metaphysical forces such as "vitalism."

Having cracked the mystery of human nutrition, Liebig went on to develop a meat extract — Liebig's Extractum Carnis — that has come down to us as bouillon and concocted the first baby formula, consisting of cow's milk, wheat flour, malted flour, and potassium bicarbonate.

Liebig, the father of modern nutritional science, had driven food into a corner and forced it to yield its chemical secrets. But the post–Liebig consensus that science now pretty much knew what was going on in food didn't last long. Doctors began to notice that many of the babies fed exclusively on Liebig's formula failed to thrive. (Not surprising, given that his preparation lacked any vitamins or several essential fats and amino acids.) That Liebig might have overlooked a few little things in food also began to occur to doctors who observed that sailors on long ocean voyages often got sick, even when they had adequate supplies of protein, carbohydrates, and fat. Clearly the chemists were missing something — some essential ingredients present in the fresh plant foods (like oranges and potatoes) that miraculously cured the sailors. This observation led to the discovery early in the twentieth century of the first set of micro-nutrients, which the Polish biochemist Casimir Funk, harkening back to older vitalist ideas of food, christened "vitamines" in 1912 ("vita-" for life and "-amines" for organic compounds organized around nitrogen).

Vitamins did a lot for the prestige of nutritional science. These special molecules, which at first were isolated from foods and then later synthesized in a laboratory, could cure people of nutritional deficiencies such as scurvy or beriberi almost overnight in a convincing demonstration of reductive chemistry's power. Beginning in the 1920s, vitamins enjoyed a vogue among the middle class, a group not notably afflicted by beriberi or scurvy. But the belief took hold that these magic molecules also promoted growth in children, long life in adults, and, in a phrase of the time, "positive health" in everyone. (And what would "negative health" be exactly?) Vitamins had brought a kind of glamour to the science of nutrition, and though certain elite segments of the population now began to eat by its expert lights, it really wasn't until late in the twentieth century that nutrients began to push food aside in the popular imagination of what it means to eat.

No single event marked the shift from eating food to eating nutrients, although in retrospect a little-noticed political dustup in Washington in 1977 seems to have helped propel American culture down this unfortunate and dimly lighted path. Responding to reports of an alarming increase in chronic diseases linked to diet — including heart disease, cancer, obesity, and diabetes — the Senate Select Committee on Nutrition and Human Needs chaired by South Dakota Senator George McGovern held hearings on the problem. The committee had been formed in 1968 with a mandate to eliminate malnutrition, and its work had led to the establishment of several important food-assistance programs. Endeavoring now to resolve the question of diet and chronic disease in the general population represented a certain amount of mission creep, but all in a good cause to which no one could possibly object.

After taking two days of testimony on diet and killer diseases, the committee's staff — comprised not of scientists or doctors but of lawyers and (ahem) journalists — set to work preparing what it had every reason to assume would be an uncontroversial document called *Dietary Goals for the United States.* The committee learned that while rates of coronary heart disease had soared in America since World War II, certain other cultures that consumed traditional diets based mostly on plants had strikingly low rates of chronic diseases. Epidemiologists had also observed that in America during the war years, when meat and dairy products were strictly rationed, the rate of heart disease had temporarily plummeted, only to leap upward once the war was over.

Beginning in the 1950s, a growing body of scientific opinion held that the consumption of fat and dietary cholesterol, much of which came from meat and dairy products, was responsible for rising rates of heart disease during the twentieth century. The "lipid hypothesis," as it was called, had already been embraced by the American Heart Association, which in 1961 had begun recommending a "prudent diet" low in saturated fat and cholesterol from animal products. True, actual proof for the lipid hypothesis was remarkably thin in 1977 — it was still very much a hypothesis, but one well on its way to general acceptance.

In January 1977, the committee issued a fairly straightforward set of dietary guidelines, calling on Americans to cut down on their consumption of red meat and dairy products. Within weeks a firestorm of criticism, emanating chiefly from the red meat and dairy industries, engulfed the committee, and Senator McGovern (who had a great many cattle ranchers among his South Dakota constituents) was forced to beat a retreat. The committee's recommendations were hastily rewritten. Plain talk about actual foodstuffs — the committee had advised Americans to "reduce consumption of meat" — was replaced by artful compromise: "choose meats, poultry, and fish that will reduce saturated fat intake."

Leave aside for now the virtues, if any, of a low-meat and/or low-fat diet, questions to which I will return, and focus for a moment on language. For with these subtle changes in wording a whole way of thinking about food and health underwent a momentous shift. First, notice that the stark message to "eat less" of a particular food — in this case meat — had been deep-sixed; don't look for it ever again in any official U.S. government dietary pronouncement. Say what you will about this or that food, you are not allowed officially to tell people to eat less of it or the industry in question will have you for lunch. But there is a path around this immovable obstacle, and it was McGovern's staffers who blazed it: *Speak no more of foods, only nutrients.* Notice how in the revised guidelines, distinctions between entities as different as beef and chicken and fish have collapsed. These three venerable foods, each representing not just a different species but an entirely different taxonomic class, are now lumped together as mere delivery systems for a single nutrient. Notice too how the new language exonerates the foods themselves. Now the culprit is an obscure, invisible, tasteless — and politically unconnected — substance that may or may not lurk in them called saturated fat.

The linguistic capitulation did nothing to rescue McGovern from his blunder. In the very next election, in 1980, the beef lobby succeeded in rusticating the three-term senator, sending an unmistakable warning to anyone who would challenge the American diet, and in particular the big chunk of animal protein squatting in the middle of its plate. Henceforth, government dietary guidelines would shun plain talk about

whole foods, each of which has its trade association on Capitol Hill, but would instead
arrive dressed in scientific euphemism and
speaking of nutrients, entities that few
Americans (including, as we would find out,
American nutrition scientists) really understood but that, with the notable exception
of sucrose, lack powerful lobbies in Washington.*

The lesson of the McGovern fiasco was
quickly absorbed by all who would pro-
nounce on the American diet. When a few

---

*Sucrose is the exception that proves the rule.
Only the power of the sugar lobby in Washington
can explain the fact that the official U.S. recommendation for the maximum permissible level of
free sugars in the diet is an eye-popping 25
percent of daily calories. To give you some idea
just how permissive that is, the World Health
Organization recommends that no more than 10
percent of daily calories come from added sugars,
a benchmark that the U.S. sugar lobby has worked
furiously to dismantle. In 2004 it enlisted the Bush
State Department in a campaign to get the recommendation changed and has threatened to lobby
Congress to cut WHO funding unless the organization recants. Perhaps we should be grateful that
the saturated fat interests have as yet organized no
such lobby.

years later the National Academy of Sciences looked into the question of diet and cancer, it was careful to frame its recommendations nutrient by nutrient rather than food by food, to avoid offending any powerful interests. We now know the academy's panel of thirteen scientists adopted this approach over the objections of at least two of its members who argued that most of the available science pointed toward conclusions about foods, not nutrients. According to T. Colin Campbell, a Cornell nutritional biochemist who served on the panel, all of the human population studies linking dietary fat to cancer actually showed that the groups with higher cancer rates consumed not just more fats, but also more animal foods and fewer plant foods as well. "This meant that these cancers could just as easily be caused by animal protein, dietary cholesterol, something else exclusively found in animal-based foods, or a lack of plant-based foods," Campbell wrote years later. The argument fell on deaf ears.

In the case of the "good foods" too, nutrients also carried the day: The language of the final report highlighted the benefits of the antioxidants in vegetables rather than the vegetables themselves. Joan Gussow, a Columbia University nutritionist who served on the panel, argued against the focus on nutrients rather than whole foods. "The really important message in the epidemiology, which is all we had to go on, was that some vegetables and citrus fruits seemed to be protective against cancer. But those sections of the report were written as though it was the vitamin C in the citrus or the beta-carotene in the vegetables that was responsible for the effect. I kept changing the language to talk about '*foods that contain* vitamin C' and '*foods that contain* carotenes.' Because how do you know it's not one of the other things in the carrots or the broccoli? There are hundreds of carotenes. But the biochemists had their answer: 'You can't do a trial on broccoli.' "

So the nutrients won out over the foods. The panel's resort to scientific reductionism had the considerable virtue of being both politically expedient (in the case of meat and dairy) and, to these scientific heirs of Justus von Liebig, intellectually sympathetic. With each of its chapters focused on a single nutrient, the final draft of the National Academy of Sciences report, *Diet, Nutrition and Cancer,* framed its recommendations in terms of saturated fats and antioxidants rather than beef and broccoli.

In doing so, the 1982 National Academy

of Sciences report helped codify the official new dietary language, the one we all still speak. Industry and media soon followed suit, and terms like *polyunsaturated, cholesterol, monounsaturated, carbohydrate, fiber, polyphenols, amino acids, flavonols, carotenoids, antioxidants, probiotics,* and *phytochemicals* soon colonized much of the cultural space previously occupied by the tangible material formerly known as food.

The Age of Nutritionism had arrived.

Two:
Nutritionism Defined

The term isn't mine. It was coined by an Australian sociologist of science by the name of Gyorgy Scrinis, and as near as I can determine first appeared in a 2002 essay titled "Sorry Marge" published in an Australian quarterly called *Meanjin.* "Sorry Marge" looked at margarine as the ultimate nutritionist product, able to shift its identity (*no cholesterol!* one year, *no trans fats!* the next) depending on the prevailing winds of dietary opinion. But Scrinis had bigger game in his sights than spreadable vegetable oil. He suggested that we look past the various nutritional claims swirling around margarine and butter and consider the underlying message of the debate itself: "namely, that we should understand and engage with food and our bodies in terms of their nutritional and chemical constituents and requirements — the assumption being that this is all we need to understand." This reductionist way of thinking about food had been pointed out and criticized before (notably by the Canadian historian Harvey Levenstein, the British nutritionist Geoffrey Cannon, and the American nutritionists Joan Gussow and Marion Nestle), but it had never before been given a proper name: "nutritionism." Proper names have a way of making visible things we don't easily see or simply take for granted.

The first thing to understand about nutritionism is that it is not the same thing as nutrition. As the "-ism" suggests, it is not a scientific subject but an ideology. Ideologies are ways of organizing large swaths of life and experience under a set of shared but unexamined assumptions. This quality makes an ideology particularly hard to see, at least while it's still exerting its hold on your culture. A reigning ideology is a little like the weather — all pervasive and so virtually impossible to escape. Still, we can try.

In the case of nutritionism, the widely shared but unexamined assumption is that the key to understanding food is indeed the nutrient. Put another way: Foods are essentially the sum of their nutrient parts. From this basic premise flow several others.

Since nutrients, as compared with foods, are invisible and therefore slightly mysterious, it falls to the scientists (and to the journalists through whom the scientists reach the public) to explain the hidden reality of foods to us. In form this is a quasireligious idea, suggesting the visible world is not the one that really matters, which implies the need for a priesthood. For to enter a world where your dietary salvation depends on unseen nutrients, you need plenty of expert help.

But expert help to do what exactly? This brings us to another unexamined assumption of nutritionism: that the whole point of eating is to maintain and promote bodily health. Hippocrates' famous injunction to "let food be thy medicine" is ritually invoked to support this notion. I'll leave the premise alone for now, except to point out that it is not shared by all cultures and, further, that the experience of these other cultures suggests that, paradoxically, regarding food as being about things other than bodily health

— like pleasure, say, or sociality or identity — makes people no less healthy; indeed, there's some reason to believe it may make them *more* healthy. This is what we usually have in mind when we speak of the French paradox. So there is at least a question as to whether the ideology of nutritionism is actually any good for you.

It follows from the premise that food is foremost about promoting physical health that the nutrients in food should be divided into the healthy ones and the unhealthy ones — good nutrients and bad. This has been a hallmark of nutritionist thinking from the days of Liebig, for whom it wasn't enough to identify the nutrients; he also had to pick favorites, and nutritionists have been doing so ever since. Liebig claimed that protein was the "master nutrient" in animal nutrition, because he believed it drove growth. Indeed, he likened the role of protein in animals to that of nitrogen in plants: Protein (which contains nitrogen) comprised the essential human fertilizer. Liebig's elevation of protein dominated nutritionist thinking for decades as public health authorities worked to expand access to and production of the master nutrient (especially in the form of animal protein), with the goal of growing bigger, and therefore (it was assumed) healthier, people. (A high priority for Western governments fighting imperial wars.) To a considerable extent we still have a food system organized around the promotion of protein as the master nutrient. It has given us, among other things, vast amounts of cheap meat and milk, which have in turn given us much, *much* bigger people. Whether they are healthier too is another question.

It seems to be a rule of nutritionism that for every good nutrient, there must be a bad nutrient to serve as its foil, the latter a focus for our food fears and the former for our enthusiasms. A backlash against protein arose in America at the turn of the last century as diet gurus like John Harvey Kellogg and Horace Fletcher (about whom more later) railed against the deleterious effects of protein on digestion (it supposedly led to the proliferation of toxic bacteria in the gut) and promoted the cleaner, more wholesome carbohydrate in its place. The legacy of that revaluation is the breakfast cereal, the strategic objective of which was to dethrone animal protein at the morning meal.

Ever since, the history of modern nutritionism has been a history of macronutrients at war: protein against carbs; carbs against proteins, and then fats; fats against carbs. Beginning with Liebig, in each age nutritionism has organized most of its energies around an imperial nutrient: protein in the nineteenth century, fat in the twentieth, and, it stands to reason, carbohydrates will occupy our attention in the twenty-first. Meanwhile, in the shadow of these titanic struggles, smaller civil wars have raged within the sprawling empires of the big three: refined carbohydrates versus fiber; animal protein versus plant protein; saturated fats versus polyunsaturated fats; and then, deep down within the province of the polyunsaturates, omega-3 fatty acids versus omega-6s. Like so many ideologies, nutritionism at bottom hinges on a form of dualism, so that at all times there must be an evil nutrient for adherents to excoriate and a savior nutrient for them to sanctify. At the moment, trans fats are performing admirably in the former role, omega-3 fatty acids in the latter. It goes without saying that such a Manichaean view of nutrition is bound to promote food fads and phobias and large abrupt swings of the nutritional pendulum.

Another potentially serious weakness of nutritionist ideology is that, focused so relentlessly as it is on the nutrients it can measure, it has trouble discerning qualitative distinctions among foods. So fish, beef, and chicken through the nutritionist's lens become mere delivery systems for varying quantities of different fats and proteins and whatever other nutrients happen to be on their scope. Milk through this lens is reduced to a suspension of protein, lactose, fats, and calcium in water, when it is entirely possible that the benefits, or for that matter the hazards, of drinking milk owe to entirely other factors (growth hormones?) or relationships between factors (fat-soluble vitamins and saturated fat?) that have been overlooked. Milk remains a food of humbling complexity, to judge by the long, sorry saga of efforts to simulate it. The entire history of baby formula has been the history of one overlooked nutrient after another: Liebig missed the vitamins and amino acids, and his successors missed the omega-3s, and still to this day babies fed on the most "nutritionally complete" formula fail to do as well as babies fed human milk. Even more than margarine, infant formula stands as the ultimate test product of nutritionism and a fair index of its hubris.

This brings us to one of the most troubling features of nutritionism, though it is a feature certainly not troubling to all. When the emphasis is on quantifying the nutrients contained in foods (or, to be precise, the *recognized* nutrients in foods), any qualitative distinction between whole foods and processed foods is apt to disappear. "[If] foods are understood only in terms of the various quantities of nutrients they contain," Gyorgy Scrinis wrote, then "even processed foods may be considered to be 'healthier' for you than whole foods if they contain the appropriate quantities of some nutrients."

How convenient.

Three: Nutritionism Comes to Market

No idea could be more sympathetic to manufacturers of processed foods, which surely explains why they have been so happy to jump on the nutritionism bandwagon. Indeed, nutritionism supplies the ultimate justification for processing food by implying that with a judicious application of food science, fake foods can be made even more nutritious than the real thing. This of course is the story of margarine, the first important synthetic food to slip into our diet. Margarine started out in the nineteenth century as a cheap and inferior substitute for butter, but with the emergence of the lipid hypothesis in the 1950s, manufacturers quickly figured out that their product, with some tinkering, could be marketed as better — smarter! — than butter: butter with the bad nutrients removed (cholesterol and saturated fats) and replaced with good nutrients (polyunsaturated fats and then vitamins). Every time margarine was found wanting, the wanted nutrient could simply be added (Vitamin D? *Got it now.* Vitamin A? *Sure, no problem*). But of course margarine, being the product not of nature but of human ingenuity, could never be any smarter than the nutritionists dictating its recipe, and the nutritionists turned out to be not nearly as smart as they thought. The food scientists' ingenious method for making healthy vegetable oil solid at room temperature — by blasting it with hydrogen — turned out to produce unhealthy trans fats, fats that we now know are more dangerous than the saturated fats they were designed to replace. Yet the beauty of a processed food like margarine is that it can be endlessly reengineered to overcome even the most embarrassing about-face in nutritional thinking — including the real wincer that its main ingredient might cause heart attacks and cancer. So now the trans fats are gone, and margarine marches on, unfazed and apparently unkillable. Too bad the same cannot be said of an unknown number of margarine eaters.

By now we have become so inured to fake foods that we forget what a difficult trail margarine had to blaze before it and other synthetic food products could win government and consumer acceptance. At least since the 1906 publication of Upton Sinclair's *The Jungle,* the "adulteration" of common foods has been a serious concern of the eating public and the target of numerous federal laws and Food and Drug Administration regulations. Many consumers regarded "oleomargarine" as just such an adulteration, and in the late 1800s five states passed laws requiring that all butter imitations be dyed pink so no one would be fooled. The Supreme Court struck down the laws in 1898. In retrospect, had the practice survived, it might have saved some lives.

The 1938 Food, Drug and Cosmetic Act imposed strict rules requiring that the word "imitation" appear on any food product that was, well, an imitation. Read today, the official rationale behind the imitation rule seems at once commonsensical and quaint: ". . . there are certain traditional foods that everyone knows, such as bread, milk and cheese, and that when consumers buy these foods, they should get the foods they are expecting . . . [and] if a food resembles a standardized food but does not comply with the standard, that food must be labeled as an 'imitation.' "

Hard to argue with that . . . but the food industry did, strenuously for decades, and in 1973 it finally succeeded in getting the imitation rule tossed out, a little-noticed but momentous step that helped speed America down the path to nutritionism.

Industry hated the imitation rule. There had been such a tawdry history of adulterated foods and related forms of snake oil in American commerce that slapping the word "imitation" on a food product was the kiss of death — an admission of adulteration and inferiority. By the 1960s and 1970s, the requirement that such a pejorative term appear on fake food packages stood in the way of innovation, indeed of the wholesale reformulation of the American food supply — a project that, in the wake of rising concerns about dietary fat and cholesterol, was coming to be seen as a good thing. What had been regarded as hucksterism and fraud in 1906 had begun to look like sound public health policy by 1973. The American

Heart Association, eager to get Americans off saturated fats and onto vegetable oils (including hydrogenated vegetable oils), was actively encouraging the food industry to "modify" various foods to get the saturated fats and cholesterol out of them, and in the early seventies the association urged that "any existing and regulatory barriers to the marketing of such foods be removed."

And so they were when, in 1973, the FDA (not, note, the Congress that wrote the law) simply repealed the 1938 rule concerning imitation foods. It buried the change in a set of new, seemingly consumer-friendly rules about nutrient labeling so that news of the imitation rule's repeal did not appear until the twenty-seventh paragraph of *The New York Times'* account, published under the headline F.D.A. PROPOSES SWEEPING CHANGE IN FOOD LABELING: NEW RULES DESIGNED TO GIVE CONSUMERS A BETTER IDEA OF NUTRITIONAL VALUE. (The second deck of the headline gave away the game: PROCESSORS BACK MOVE.) The revised imitation rule held that as long as an imitation product was not "nutritionally inferior" to the natural food it sought to impersonate — as long as it had the same quantities of recognized nutrients — the imitation could be marketed without using the dreaded "i" word.

With that, the regulatory door was thrown open to all manner of faked low-fat products: Fats in things like sour cream and yogurt could now be replaced with hydrogenated oils or guar gum or carrageenan, bacon bits could be replaced with soy protein, the cream in "whipped cream" and "coffee creamer" could be replaced with corn starch, and the yolks of liquefied eggs could be replaced with, well, whatever the food scientists could dream up, because the sky was now the limit. As long as the new fake foods were engineered to be nutritionally equivalent to the real article, they could no longer be considered fake. Of course the operative nutritionist assumption here is that we know enough to determine nutritional equivalence — something that the checkered history of baby formula suggests has never been the case.

Nutritionism had become the official ideology of the Food and Drug Administration; for all practical purposes the government had redefined foods as nothing more than the sum of their recognized nutrients. Adulteration had been repositioned as food science. All it would take now was a push from McGovern's *Dietary Goals* for hundreds of "traditional foods that everyone knows" to begin their long retreat from the supermarket shelves and for our eating to become more "scientific."

Four:
Food Science's Golden Age

In the years following the 1977 *Dietary Goals* and the 1982 National Academy of Sciences report on diet and cancer, the food industry, armed with its regulatory absolution, set about reengineering thousands of popular food products to contain more of the nutrients that science and government had deemed the good ones and fewer of the bad. A golden age for food science dawned. Hyphens sprouted like dandelions in the supermarket aisles: *low-fat, no-cholesterol, high-fiber.* Ingredients labels on formerly two- or three-ingredient foods such as mayonnaise and bread and yogurt ballooned with lengthy lists of new additives — what in a more benighted age would have been called adulterants. The Year of Eating Oat Bran — also known as 1988 — served as a kind of coming-out party for the food scientists, who succeeded in getting the material into nearly every processed food sold in America. Oat bran's moment on the dietary stage didn't last long, but the pattern now was set, and every few years since then, a new oat bran has taken its star turn under the marketing lights. (Here come omega-3s!)

You would not think that common food animals could themselves be rejiggered to fit nutritionist fashion, but in fact some of them could be, and were, in response to the 1977 and 1982 dietary guidelines as animal scientists figured out how to breed leaner pigs and select for leaner beef. With widespread lipophobia taking hold of the human population, countless cattle lost their marbling and lean pork was repositioned as "the new white meat" — tasteless and tough as running shoes, perhaps, but now even a pork chop could compete with chicken as a way for eaters to "reduce saturated fat intake." In the years since then, egg producers figured out a clever way to redeem even the disreputable egg: By feeding flaxseed to hens, they could elevate levels of omega-3 fatty acids in the yolks. Aiming to do the same thing for pork and beef fat, the animal scientists are now at work genetically engineering omega-3 fatty acids into pigs and persuading cattle to lunch on flaxseed in the hope of introducing the blessed fish fat where it had never gone before: into hot dogs and hamburgers.

But these whole foods are the exceptions. The typical whole food has much more trouble competing under the rules of nutritionism, if only because something like a banana or an avocado can't quite as readily change its nutritional stripes. (Though rest assured the genetic engineers are hard at work on the problem.) To date, at least, they can't put oat bran in a banana or omega-3s in a peach. So depending on the reigning nutritional orthodoxy, the avocado might either be a high-fat food to be assiduously avoided (Old Think) or a food high in monounsaturated fat to be embraced (New Think). The fate and supermarket sales of each whole food rises and falls with every change in the nutritional weather while the processed foods simply get reformulated and differently supplemented. That's why when the Atkins diet storm hit the food industry in 2003, bread and pasta got a quick redesign (dialing back the carbs; boosting the proteins) while poor unreconstructed potatoes and carrots were left out in the carbohydrate cold. (The low-carb indignities visited on bread and pasta, two formerly "traditional foods that everyone knows," would never have been possible had the imitation rule not been tossed out in

1973. Who would ever buy imitation spaghetti? But of course that is precisely what low-carb pasta is.)

A handful of lucky whole foods have recently gotten the "good nutrient" marketing treatment: The antioxidants in the pomegranate (a fruit formerly more trouble to eat than it was worth) now protect against cancer and erectile dysfunction, apparently, and the omega-3 fatty acids in the (formerly just fattening) walnut ward off heart disease. A whole subcategory of nutritional science — funded by industry and, according to one recent analysis,* remarkably reliable in its ability to find a health benefit in whatever food it has been commissioned to study — has sprung up to give a nutritionist sheen — (and FDA-approved health claim) to all sorts of foods, including some not ordinarily thought of as healthy. The Mars Corporation recently endowed a chair in chocolate science at the University of California at Davis, where

*L. I. Lesser, C. B. Ebbeling, M. Goozner, D. Wypij, and D. S. Ludwig, "Relationship Between Funding Source and Conclusion Among Nutrition-Related Scientific Articles," *PLoS Medicine,* Vol. 4, No. 1, e5 doi:10.1371/journal.pmed .0040005.

research on the antioxidant properties of cacao is making breakthroughs, so it shouldn't be long before we see chocolate bars bearing FDA-approved health claims. (When we do, nutritionism will surely have entered its baroque phase.) Fortunately for everyone playing this game, scientists can find an antioxidant in just about any plant-based food they choose to study.

Yet as a general rule it's a whole lot easier to slap a health claim on a box of sugary cereal than on a raw potato or a carrot, with the perverse result that the most healthful foods in the supermarket sit there quietly in the produce section, silent as stroke victims, while a few aisles over in Cereal the Cocoa Puffs and Lucky Charms are screaming their newfound "whole-grain goodness" to the rafters.

Watch out for those health claims.

FIVE:
THE MELTING OF THE LIPID HYPOTHESIS

Nutritionism is good for the food business. But is it good for us? You might think that a national fixation on nutrients would lead to measurable improvements in public health.

For that to happen, however, the underlying nutritional science and the policy recommendations (not to mention the journalism) based on that science would both have to be sound. This has seldom been the case.

The most important such nutrition campaign has been the thirty-year effort to reform the food supply and our eating habits in light of the lipid hypothesis — the idea that dietary fat is responsible for chronic disease. At the behest of government panels, nutrition scientists, and public health officials, we have dramatically changed the way we eat and the way we think about food, in what stands as the biggest experiment in applied nutritionism in history. Thirty years later, we have good reason to believe that putting the nutritionists in charge of the menu and the kitchen has not only ruined an untold number of meals, but also has done little for our health, except very possibly to make it worse.

These are strong words, I know. Here are a couple more: What the Soviet Union was to the ideology of Marxism, the Low-Fat Campaign is to the ideology of nutritionism — its supreme test and, as now is coming clear, its most abject failure. You can argue, as some diehards will do, that the problem was one of faulty execution or you can accept that the underlying tenets of the ideology contained the seeds of the eventual disaster.

At this point you're probably saying to yourself, *Hold on just a minute. Are you really saying the whole low-fat deal was bogus? But my supermarket is still packed with low-fat this and no-cholesterol that! My doctor is still on me about my cholesterol and telling me to switch to low-fat everything.* I was flabbergasted at the news too, because no one in charge — not in the government, not in the public health community — has dared to come out and announce: *Um, you know everything we've been telling you for the last thirty years about the links between dietary fat and heart disease? And fat and cancer? And fat and fat? Well, this just in: It now appears that none of it was true. We sincerely regret the error.*

No, the admissions of error have been muffled, and the mea culpas impossible to find. But read around in the recent scientific literature and you will find a great many scientists beating a quiet retreat from the main tenets of the lipid hypothesis. Let me offer just one example, an article from a group of prominent nutrition scientists at the Harvard School of Public Health. In a recent review of the relevant research called

"Types of Dietary Fat and Risk of Coronary Heart Disease: A Critical Review,"[*] the authors proceed to calmly remove, one by one, just about every strut supporting the theory that dietary fat causes heart disease.

Hu and his colleagues begin with a brief, uninflected summary of the lipophobic era that is noteworthy mostly for casting the episode in the historical past:

> During the past several decades, reduction in fat intake has been the main focus of national dietary recommendations. In the public's mind, the words "dietary fat" have become synonymous with obesity and heart disease, whereas the words "low-fat" and "fat-free" have been synonymous with heart health.

We can only wonder how in the world such crazy ideas ever found their way into the "public's mind." Surely not from anyone associated with the Harvard School of Public Health, I would hope. Well, as it turns out, the selfsame group, formerly in thrall to the lipid hypothesis, was recommending until the early 1990s, when the evidence about the dangers of trans fats

*Frank B. Hu, et al., *Journal of the American College of Nutrition,* Vol. 20, 1, 5–19 (2001).

could no longer be ignored, that people reduce their saturated fat intake by switching from butter to margarine. (Though red flags about trans fats can be spotted as far back as 1956, when Ancel Keyes, the father of the lipid hypothesis, suggested that rising consumption of hydrogenated vegetable oils might be responsible for the twentieth-century rise in coronary heart disease.)

But back to the critical review, which in its second paragraph drops this bombshell:

It is now increasingly recognized that the low-fat campaign has been based on little scientific evidence and may have caused unintended health consequences.

Say what?

The article then goes on blandly to survey the crumbling foundations of the lipid hypothesis, circa 2001: Only two studies have ever found "a significant positive association between saturated fat intake and risk of CHD [coronary heart disease]"; many more have failed to find an association. Only one study has ever found "a significant inverse association between polyunsaturated fat intake and CHD." Let me translate: The amount of saturated fat in the diet probably may have little if any bearing on the risk of heart disease, and evidence that increasing polyunsaturated fats in the diet will reduce risk is slim to nil. As for the dangers of dietary cholesterol, the review found "a weak and nonsignificant positive association between dietary cholesterol and risk of CHD." (Someone should tell the food processors, who continue to treat dietary cholesterol as a matter of life and death.) "Surprisingly," the authors wrote, "there is little direct evidence linking higher egg consumption and increased risk of CHD" — surprising, because eggs are particularly high in cholesterol.

By the end of the review, there *is* one strong association between a type of dietary fat and heart disease left standing, and it happens to be precisely the type of fat that the low-fat campaigners have spent most of the last thirty years encouraging us to consume more of: trans fats. It turns out that "a higher intake of *trans* fat can contribute to increased risk of CHD through multiple mechanisms"; to wit, it raises bad cholesterol and lowers good cholesterol (something not even the evil saturated fats can do); it increases triglycerides, a risk factor for CHD; it promotes inflammation and possibly thrombogenesis (clotting), and it may promote insulin resistance. Trans fat is *really* bad stuff, apparently, fully twice as bad as saturated fat in its impact on cholesterol ratios. If any of the authors of the critical review are conscious of the cosmic irony here — that the principal contribution of thirty years of official nutritional advice has been to replace a possibly mildly unhealthy fat in our diets with a demonstrably lethal one — they are not saying.

The paper is not quite prepared to throw out the entire lipid hypothesis, but by the end precious little of it is left standing. The authors conclude that while total levels of fat in the diet apparently have little bearing on the risk of heart disease (!), the ratio between types of fats does. Adding omega-3 fatty acids to the diet (that is, eating *more* of a certain kind of fat) "substantially reduces coronary and total mortality" in heart patients, and replacing saturated fats with polyunsaturated fats lowers blood cholesterol, which they deem an important risk factor for CHD. (Some researchers no longer do, pointing out that half the people who get heart attacks don't have elevated cholesterol levels, and about half the people with elevated cholesterol do not suffer from CHD.) One other little grenade is dropped in the paper's conclusion: Although "a major purported benefit of a low-fat diet is weight loss," a review of the literature failed to turn up any convincing evidence of this proposition. To the contrary, it found "some evidence" that replacing fats in the diet with carbohydrates (as official dietary advice has urged us to do since the 1970s) *will* lead to weight gain.

I have dwelled on this paper because it fairly reflects the current thinking on the increasingly tenuous links between dietary fat and health. The lipid hypothesis is quietly melting away, but no one in the public health community, or the government, seems quite ready to publicly acknowledge it. For fear of what exactly? That we'll binge on bacon double cheeseburgers? More likely that we'll come to the unavoidable conclusion that the emperors of nutrition have no clothes and never listen to them again.

In fact, there have been dissenters to the lipid hypothesis all along, lipid biochemists like Mary Enig (who has been sounding the alarm on trans fats since the 1970s) and nutritionists like Fred Kummerow and John Yudkin (who have been sounding the alarm on refined carbohydrates, also since the 1970s), but these critics have always had trouble getting a hearing, especially after 1977, when the McGovern guidelines effectively closed off debate on the lipid hypothesis.

Scientific paradigms are never easy to challenge, even when they begin to crack under the weight of contradictory evidence. Few scientists ever look back to see where they and their paradigms might have gone astray; rather, they're trained to keep moving forward, doing yet more science to add to the increments of our knowledge, patching up and preserving whatever of the current consensus can be preserved until the next big idea comes along. So don't count on a scientific Aleksandr Solzhenitsyn to show up and expose the whole fat paradigm as a historical disaster.

The closest thing to such a figure we have had is not a scientist but a science journalist named Gary Taubes, who for the last decade has been blowing the whistle on the science behind the low-fat campaign. In a devastating series of articles and an important new book called *Good Calories, Bad Calories,* Taubes has all but demolished the whole lipid hypothesis, demonstrating just how little scientific backing it had from the very beginning.

Indeed. Wind the tape back to 1976, and you find plenty of reasons to doubt the lipid hypothesis even then. Some of these reasons were circumstantial, but nevertheless compelling. For instance, during the decades of the twentieth century when rates of heart disease were rising in America, Americans were actually *reducing* their intake of animal fats (in the form of lard and tallow). In place of those fats, they consumed substantially more vegetable oils, especially in the form of margarine, sales of which outpaced butter for the first time in 1957. Between the end of World War II and 1976 (the year of McGovern's hearings), per capita consumption of animal fats from all sources dropped from eighty-four pounds to seventy-one, while fats from seed oils approximately doubled. Americans appeared to be moving in the direction of a "prudent diet" and yet, paradoxically, having more heart attacks on it, not fewer.[*]

As for the precipitous decline in heart disease during the years of World War II, that could just as easily be attributed to factors other than the scarcity of meat, butter,

---

[*]In 1945, 217,000 deaths in the United States were attributed to heart attacks. By 1960 there were 500,000. By 2001 that number had fallen to 185,000. (It's important to note that the diagnostic criteria for heart attack have changed over time, as has the size of the population.)

and eggs. Not just animal protein, but sugar and gasoline were also strictly rationed during the war. Americans generally ate less of everything, including, notably, refined carbohydrates; they did, however, eat more fish. And got more exercise because they couldn't drive as freely thanks to gas rationing.

But the lipid hypothesis would not be deterred. Researchers in the 1950s and 1960s had studied populations in other countries that had substantially lower rates of heart disease, which could be explained by their lower consumption of saturated fat. That it could just as easily be explained by other factors — fewer total calories? fewer refined carbohydrates? more exercise? more fruits and vegetables or fish? — did not disturb the gathering consensus that fat must be the key.

The consensus hinged on two suggestive links that were well established by the early sixties: a link between high rates of cholesterol in the blood and the likelihood of heart disease and a link between saturated fat in the diet and cholesterol levels in the blood. Both these links have held up, but it doesn't necessarily follow from them that consumption of saturated fat leads to heart disease, unless you can also demonstrate that serum cholesterol is a cause of heart disease and not, say, just a symptom of it. And though evidence for a link between cholesterol in the diet and cholesterol in the blood has always been tenuous, the belief that the former contributed to the latter has persisted, perhaps because it makes such intuitive sense — and perhaps because it has been so heavily promoted by the margarine makers.

Despite these gaps, it seemed a short easy step for McGovern's committee to link the links, as it were, and conclude that eating meat and dairy (as important sources of both saturated fat and cholesterol) contributed to heart disease. After all, the American Heart Association had already taken the same short link-linking step and had been advocating a prudent diet low in fat and cholesterol since 1961. Still, the committee was not unaware of the controversy surrounding the research on which it was basing its recommendations. It had received a strongly worded letter of dissent from the American Medical Association, arguing that "there is a potential for harmful effects for a radical long-term dietary change as would occur through adoption of the proposed national goal."

Still, the national goal was adopted. Never

before had the government endeavored to change the diet of the whole population. In the past nutritional policies had targeted particular populations at risk for particular deficiencies. But as Taubes has documented, the attitude on the committee was that even if all the data weren't hard as rock quite yet, what would be the harm in getting Americans to cut down on dietary fats? At the press conference introducing the *Dietary Goals,* Mark Hegsted, the Harvard School of Public Health nutritionist who helped to shape them, put it this way: "The question to be asked is not why we should change our diet, but why not?"

At least one good answer to that question was apparently overlooked. Perhaps because fat was in such bad repute in 1977, Dr. Hegsted and his colleagues must not have stopped to consider how a change in the levels or ratios of the various lipids, and the promotion of a biologically novel fat like trans fat, might affect human physiology. It bears remembering that the human brain is about 60 percent fat; every neuron is sheathed in a protective layer of the stuff. Fats make up the structure of our cell walls, the ratios between the various kinds influencing the permeability of the cells to everything from glucose and hormones to microbes and toxins. Without adequate amounts of fat in the diet, fat-soluble vitamins like A and E can't pass through the intestinal walls. All this was known in 1977. But the Hippocratic oath — "First do no harm" — evidently does not apply to official dietary advice, which at least in 1977 followed a very different principle: "Why not?"

So potentially much was at stake for our health and well-being when the government threw its weight behind a wholesale change in the American diet. True, it was entirely possible that the nation would have chosen simply to ignore the *Dietary Goals* and go on eating as it had. But that's not what happened. Instead, the goals were taken seriously, and one of the more ambitious nutritional experiments in our history got under way. Authority over the national menu, which in the past had rested largely with tradition and habit (and mom), shifted perceptibly in January 1977: Culture ceded a large measure of its influence over how we ate and thought about eating to science. Or what passes for science in dietary matters; nutritionism would be a more accurate term. "Premature or not," *The New York Times'* Jane Brody wrote in 1981, "the *Dietary Goals* are beginning to reshape the nutritional philosophy, if not yet the eating habits, of most Americans."

SIX:
EAT RIGHT, GET FATTER

In fact, we did change our eating habits in the wake of the new guidelines, endeavoring to replace the evil fats at the top of the food pyramid with the good carbs spread out at the bottom. The whole of the industrial food supply was reformulated to reflect the new nutritional wisdom, giving us low-fat pork, low-fat Snackwell's, and all the low-fat pasta and high-fructose (yet low-fat!) corn syrup we could consume. Which turned out to be quite a lot. Oddly, Americans got really fat on their new low-fat diet — indeed, many date the current epidemic of obesity and diabetes to the late 1970s, when Americans began bingeing on carbohydrates, ostensibly as a way to avoid the evils of fat.

But the story is slightly more complicated than that. For while it is true that Americans post–1977 did shift the balance in their diets from fats to carbs so that *fat as a percentage of total calories* in the diet declined (from 42 percent in 1977 to 34 percent in 1995), we never did in fact cut down on our total consumption of fat; we just ate more of other things. We did reduce our consumption of saturated fats, replacing them, as directed, with polyunsaturated fats and trans fats. Meat consumption actually held steady, though we did, again as instructed, shift from red meat to white to reduce our saturated fat intake. Basically what we did was heap a bunch more carbs onto our plate, obscuring but by no means replacing the expanding chunk of (now skinless white) animal protein still sitting there in the middle.

How did *that* happen? I would submit that the ideology of nutritionism deserves as much of the blame as the carbohydrates themselves do — that and human nature. By framing dietary advice in terms of good and bad nutrients, and by burying the recommendation that we should eat less of any particular actual food, it was easy for the take-home message of the 1977 and 1982 dietary guidelines to be simplified as follows: *Eat more low-fat foods.* And that is precisely what we did. We're always happy to receive a dispensation to eat more of *some*thing (with the possible exception of oat bran), and one of the things nutritionism reliably gives us is some such dispensation: low-fat cookies then, low-carb beer now. It's hard to imagine the low-fat/high-carb craze taking off as it did or our collective health deteriorating to the extent that it has if McGovern's original food-based recommendation had stood: *Eat less meat and fewer dairy products.* For how do you get from that stark counsel to the idea that another carton of Snackwell's is just what the doctor ordered?

You begin to see how attractive nutritionism is for all parties concerned, consumers as well as producers, not to mention the nutrition scientists and journalists it renders indispensable. The ideology offers a respectable rationale for creating and marketing all manner of new processed foods and permission for people to eat them. Plus, every course correction in nutritionist advice gives reason to write new diet books and articles, manufacture a new line of products, and eat a whole bunch of even more healthy new food products. And if a product is healthy by design and official sanction, then eating *lots* of it must be healthy too — maybe even more so.

Nutritionism might be the best thing ever to happen to the food industry, which historically has labored under the limits to growth imposed by a population of eaters that isn't expanding nearly as fast as the food makers need it to if they are to satisfy the expectations of Wall Street. Nutritionism solves the problem of the fixed stomach, as it used to be called in the business: the fact that compared to other consumer products, demand for food has in the past been fairly inelastic. People could eat only so much, and because tradition and habit ruled their choices, they tended to eat the same old things. Not anymore! Not only does nutritionism favor ever more novel kinds of highly processed foods (which are by far the most profitable kind to make), it actually enlists the medical establishment and the government in the promotion of those products. Play your cards right and you can even get the American Heart Association to endorse your new breakfast cereal as "heart healthy." As I write, the FDA has just signed off on a new health claim for Frito-Lay chips on the grounds that eating chips fried in polyunsaturated fats can help you reduce your consumption of saturated fats, thereby conferring blessings on your cardiovascular system. So can a notorious junk food pass through the needle eye of nutritionist logic and come out the other side looking like a health food.

SEVEN:
BEYOND THE PLEASURE PRINCIPLE

We eaters, alas, don't reap nearly as much benefit from nutritionism as food producers. Beyond providing a license to eat more of the latest approved foodlike substance, which we surely do appreciate, nutritionism tends to foster a great deal of anxiety around the experience of shopping for food and eating it. To do it right, you've got to be up on the latest scientific research, study ever-longer and more confusing ingredients labels,[*] sift through increasingly dubious health claims, and then attempt to enjoy foods that have been engineered with many other objectives in view than simply tasting good. To think of some of the most delicious components of food as toxins, as nutritionism has taught us to do in the case of fat, does little for our happiness as eaters. Americans have embraced a "nutritional philosophy," to borrow Jane Brody's words,

[*]Geoffrey Cannon points out that nutrition labels, which have become the single most ubiquitous medium of chemical information in our lives, "are advertisements for the chemical principle of nutrition."

that, regardless of whether that philosophy does anything for our health, surely takes much of the pleasure out of eating.

But why do we even need a nutritional philosophy in the first place? Perhaps because we Americans have always had a problem taking pleasure in eating. We certainly have gone to unusual lengths to avoid it. Harvey Levenstein, who has written two illuminating histories of American food culture, suggests that the sheer abundance of food in America has bred "a vague indifference to food, manifested in a tendency to eat and run, rather than to dine and savor." To savor food, to conceive of a meal as an aesthetic experience, has been regarded as evidence of effeteness, a form of foreign foppery. (Few things have been more likely to get an American political candidate in hot water than a taste for fine food, as Martin Van Buren discovered during his failed 1840 reelection campaign. Van Buren had brought a French chef to the White House, a blunder seized on by his opponent, William Henry Harrison, who made much of the fact that *he* subsisted on "raw beef and salt." George H. W. Bush's predilection for pork rinds and Bill Clinton's for Big Macs were politically astute tastes to show off.)

It could well be that, as Levenstein contends, the sheer abundance of food in America has fostered a culture of careless, perfunctory eating. But our Puritan roots also impeded a sensual or aesthetic enjoyment of food. Like sex, the need to eat links us to the animals, and historically a great deal of Protestant energy has gone into helping us keep all such animal appetites under strict control. To the Christian social reformers of the nineteenth century, "The naked act of eating was little more than unavoidable . . . and was not to be considered a pleasure except with great discretion." I'm quoting from Laura Shapiro's *Perfection Salad,* which recounts the campaign of these domestic reformers to convince Americans, in the words of one, "that eating is something more than animal indulgence, and that cooking has a nobler purpose than the gratification of appetite and the sense of taste." And what might that nobler purpose be? Sound nutrition and good sanitation. By elevating those scientific principles and "disdaining the proof of the palate," Shapiro writes, "they made it possible for American cooking to accept a flood of damaging innovations for years to come" — low-fat processed food products prominent among them.

So scientific eating is an old and venerable tradition in America. Here's how Harvey Levenstein sums up the quasiscientific beliefs that have shaped American attitudes toward food for more than a century: "that taste is not a true guide to what should be eaten; that one should not simply eat what one enjoys; that the important components of foods cannot be seen or tasted, but are discernible only in scientific laboratories; and that experimental science has produced rules of nutrition which will prevent illness and encourage longevity." Levenstein could be describing the main tenets of nutritionism.

Perhaps the most notorious flowering of pseudoscientific eating (and proto-nutritionism) came in the early years of the twentieth century, when John Harvey Kellogg and Horace Fletcher persuaded thousands of Americans to trade all pleasure in eating for health-promoting dietary regimens of truly breathtaking rigor and perversity. The two diet gurus were united in their contempt for animal protein, the consumption of which Dr. Kellogg, a Seventh-Day Adventist who bore a striking resemblance to KFC's Colonel Sanders, firmly believed promoted both masturbation and the proliferation of toxic bacteria in the colon. During this, the first golden age of American food faddism, protein performed much the same role that fat would perform during the next. At Kellogg's Battle Creek sanitarium, patients (who included John D. Rockefeller and Theodore Roosevelt) paid a small fortune to be subjected to such "scientific" practices as hourly yogurt enemas (to undo the damage that protein supposedly wreaked on the colon); electrical stimulation and "massive vibration" of the abdomen; diets consisting of nothing but grapes (ten to fourteen pounds of them a day); and at every meal, "Fletcherizing," the practice of chewing each bite of food approximately one hundred times. (Often to the rousing accompaniment of special chewing songs.) The theory was that thorough mastication would reduce protein intake (this seems certain) and thereby improve "subjective and objective well-being." Horace Fletcher (aka "the great masticator") had no scientific credentials whatsoever, but the example of his own extraordinary fitness — at fifty he could bound up and down the Washington Monument's 898 steps without pausing to catch his breath — while existing on a daily regimen of only 45 well-chewed grams of protein was all the proof his adherents needed.* The brothers Henry and William James both became enthusiastic "chewers."†

Whatever their biological efficacy, all these dietary exertions had the effect of removing eating from social life and pleasure from eating; compulsive chewing (much less hourly enema breaks) is not exactly conducive to the pleasures of the table. Also, Fletcherizing would have forcibly drained food of the very last glimmer of flavor long before the hundredth contraction of the jaw had been counted. Kellogg himself was outspoken in his hostility to the pleasures of eating: "The decline of a nation commences when gourmandizing begins."

*According to Levenstein, scientists seeking the secret of Fletcher's exemplary health scrupulously monitored his ingestions and excretions, "noting with regard to the latter, as all observers did, the remarkable absence of odor" (Levenstein, *Revolution of the Table*, p. 89).

†William James wrote of Fletcher that "if his observations on diet, confirmed already on a limited scale, should prove true on a universal scale, it is impossible to overestimate their revolutionary import." Fletcher returned the favor, assuring the philosopher that Fletcherism was "advancing the same cause as Pragmatism" (Levenstein, *Revolution of the Table*, p. 92).

If that is so, America had little reason to worry.

America's early attraction to various forms of scientific eating may also have reflected discomfort about the way other people eat: the weird, messy, smelly, and mixed-up eating habits of immigrants.* How a people eats is one of the most powerful ways they have to express, and preserve, their cultural identity, which is exactly what you *don't* want in a society dedicated to the ideal of "Americanization." To make food choices more scientific is to empty them of their ethnic content and history; in theory, at least, nutritionism proposes a neutral, modernist, forward-looking, and potentially unifying answer to the question of what it might mean to eat like an American. It is also a way to moralize about other people's choices without seeming to. In this, nutri-

---

*Americans were particularly disturbed by the way many immigrant groups mixed their foods in stews and such, in contrast to the Anglo-American practice of keeping foods separate on the plate, the culinary format anthropologist Mary Douglas calls "1A plus 2B" — one chunk of animal protein plus two vegetables or starches. Perhaps the disdain for mixing foods reflected anxieties about other kinds of mixing.

tionism is a little like the institution of the American front lawn, an unobjectionable, if bland, way to pave over our differences and Americanize the landscape. Of course in both cases unity comes at the price of aesthetic diversity and sensory pleasure. Which may be precisely the point.

EIGHT:
THE PROOF IN THE LOW-FAT PUDDING

Whatever the sacrifice of pleasure, it would be made up for by better health — that, at least, has always been nutritionism's promise. But it's difficult to conclude that scientific eating has contributed to our health. As mentioned, the low-fat campaign coincided with a dramatic increase in the incidence of obesity and diabetes in America. You could blame this unfortunate fallout on us eaters for following the official advice to eat more low-fat food a little too avidly. This explanation suggests that the problem with the low-fat campaign has been in its execution rather than in the theory behind it, and that a better, clearer public health message might have saved us from ourselves. But it is also possible that the advice itself, to replace fats in the diet with carbohydrates, was misguided. As the Hu paper suggests, there is a growing body of evidence that shifting from fats to carbohydrates may lead to weight gain (as well as a host of other problems). This is counterintuitive, because fats contain nearly twice as many calories as carbs (9 per gram for fats as compared to 5 for either carbohydrates or protein). The theory is that refined carbohydrates interfere with insulin metabolism in ways that increase hunger and promote overeating and fat storage in the body. (Call it the carbohydrate hypothesis; it's coming.)[*] If this is

[*]Gary Taubes describes the developing carbohydrate hypothesis at great length in *Good Calories, Bad Calories.* According to the hypothesis, most of the damage to our health that has been wrongly attributed to fats for the past half century — heart disease, obesity, cancer, diabetes, and so on — can rightly be blamed on refined carbohydrates. But the healthy skepticism Taubes brought to the lipid hypothesis is nowhere in evidence when he writes about the (also unproven) carbohydrate hypothesis. Even if refined carbohydrates do represent a more serious threat to health than dietary fat, to dwell on any one nutrient to the exclusion of all others is to commit the same reductionist error that the lipophobes did. Indeed,

true, then there is no escaping the conclusion that the dietary advice enshrined not only in the McGovern "Goals" but also in the National Academy of Sciences report, the dietary guidelines of the American Heart Association and the American Cancer Society and the U.S. food pyramid bears direct responsibility for creating the public health crisis that now confronts us.

Even if we accept the epidemic of obesity and diabetes as the unintended consequence of the war against dietary fat — collateral damage, you might say — what about the intended consequence of that campaign: the reduction of heart disease? Here is where the low-fat campaigners have chosen to make their last stand, pointing proudly to the fact that after peaking in the late sixties,

---

Taubes is so single-minded in his demonization of the carbohydrate that he overlooks several other possible explanations for the deleterious effects of the Western diet, including deficiencies of omega-3s and micronutrients from plants. He also downplays the risks (to health as well as eating pleasure) of the high-protein Atkins diet that the carbohydrate hypothesis implies is a sound way to eat. As its title suggests, *Good Calories, Bad Calories,* valuable as it is, does not escape the confines of nutritionism.

deaths from heart disease fell dramatically in America, a 50 percent decline since 1969. Cholesterol levels have also fallen. Epidemiologist Walter C. Willett of the Harvard School of Public Health (a coauthor of the Hu paper) cites the increase in consumption of polyunsaturated fats "as a major factor, if not the most important factor, in the decline in heart disease" observed in the seventies and eighties and calls the campaign to replace saturated fats in the diet one of the great public health success stories of our time. And so it would appear to be: We reduced our saturated fat intake, our cholesterol levels fell, and many fewer people dropped dead of heart attacks.

Whether the low-fat campaigners should take the credit for this achievement is doubtful, however. Reducing mortality from heart disease is not the same thing as reducing the incidence of heart disease, and there's reason to question whether underlying rates of heart disease have greatly changed in the last thirty years, as they should have if changes in diet were so important. A ten-year study of heart disease mortality published in the *New England Journal of Medicine* in 1998 strongly suggests that most of the decline in deaths from heart disease is due not to changes in lifestyle, such as diet, but to improvements in medical care. (Though cessation of smoking has been important.) For while during the period under analysis, heart attack deaths declined substantially, hospital admissions for heart attack did not. Modern medicine is clearly saving more people suffering from heart disease, but it appears that we haven't had nearly as much success eliminating the disease itself.

NINE:
BAD SCIENCE

To understand how nutrition science could have been so spectacularly wrong about dietary fat and health, it's important to understand that doing nutrition science isn't easy. In fact, it's a lot harder than most of the scientists who do it for a living realize or at least are willing to admit. For one thing, the scientific tools at their disposal are in many ways ill suited to the task of understanding systems as complex as food and diet. The assumptions of nutritionism — such as the idea that a food is not a system but rather the sum of its nutrient parts — pose another set of problems. We like to think of scientists as being free from ideological taint, but of course they are as much the product of their ideological environment as the rest of us. In the same way nutritionism can lead to a false consciousness in the mind of the eater, it can just as easily mislead the scientist.

The problem starts with the nutrient. Most nutritional science involves studying one nutrient at a time, a seemingly unavoidable approach that even nutritionists who do it will tell you is deeply flawed. "The problem with nutrient-by-nutrient nutrition science," points out Marion Nestle, a New York University nutritionist, "is that it takes the nutrient out of the context of the food, the food out of the context of the diet, and the diet out of the context of the lifestyle."

If nutrition scientists know this, why do they do it anyway? Because a nutrient bias is built into the way science is done. Scientists study variables they can isolate; if they can't isolate a variable, they won't be able to tell whether its presence or absence is meaningful. Yet even the simplest food is a hopelessly complicated thing to analyze, a virtual wilderness of chemical compounds, many of which exist in intricate and dynamic relation to one another, and all of which together are in the process of changing from one state to another. So if you're a nutrition scientist you do the only thing you *can* do, given the tools at your disposal: Break the thing down into its component parts and study those one by one, even if that means ignoring subtle interactions and contexts and the fact that the whole may well be more than, or maybe just different from, the sum of its parts. This is what we mean by reductionist science.

Scientific reductionism is an undeniably powerful tool, but it can mislead us too, especially when applied to something as complex, on the one side, as a food and on the other a human eater. It encourages us to take a simple mechanistic view of that transaction: Put in this nutrient, get out that physiological result. Yet people differ in important ways. We all know that lucky soul who can eat prodigious quantities of fattening food without ever gaining weight. Some populations can metabolize sugars better than others. Depending on your evolutionary heritage, you may or may not be able to digest the lactose in milk. Depending on your genetic makeup, reducing the saturated fat in your diet may or may not move your cholesterol numbers. The specific ecology of your intestines helps determine how efficiently you digest what you eat, so that the same 100 calories of food may yield more or less food energy depending on the proportion of Firmicutes and Bacteroides resident in your gut. In turn, that balance of bacterial species could owe to your genes or to something in your environment. So there is nothing very machinelike about the human eater, and to think of food as simply fuel is to completely misconstrue it. It's worth keeping in mind too that, curiously, the human digestive tract has roughly as many neurons as the spinal column. We don't yet know exactly what they're up to, but their existence suggests that much more is going on in digestion than simply the breakdown of foods into chemicals.

Also, people don't eat nutrients; they eat foods, and foods can behave very differently from the nutrients they contain. Based on epidemiological comparisons of different populations, researchers have long believed that a diet containing lots of fruits and vegetables confers some protection against cancer. So naturally they ask, What nutrient in those plant foods is responsible for that effect? One hypothesis is that the antioxidants in fresh produce — compounds like beta-carotene, lycopene, vitamin E, and so on — are the X factor. It makes good theoretical sense: These molecules (which plants produce to protect themselves from the highly reactive forms of oxygen they produce during photosynthesis) soak up the free radicals in our bodies, which can damage DNA and initiate cancers. At least that's how it seems to work in a test tube. Yet as soon as you remove these crucial molecules from the context of the whole foods they're found in, as we've done in creating antioxidant supplements, they don't seem to work at all. Indeed, in the case of beta-carotene ingested as a supplement, one study has suggested that in some people it may actually *increase* the risk of certain cancers. Big oops.

What's going on here? We don't know. It could be the vagaries of human digestion. Maybe the fiber (or some other component) in a carrot protects the antioxidant molecule from destruction by stomach acids early in the digestive process. Or it could be we isolated the wrong antioxidant. Beta is just one of a whole slew of carotenes found in common vegetables; maybe we focused on the wrong one. Or maybe beta-carotene works as an antioxidant only in concert with some other plant chemical or process; under other circumstances it may behave as a pro-oxidant.

Indeed, to look at the chemical composition of any common food plant is to realize just how much complexity lurks within it.

Here's a list of just the antioxidants that have been identified in a leaf of garden-variety thyme:

alanine, anethole essential oil, apigenin, ascorbic acid, beta-carotene, caffeic acid, camphene, carvacrol, chlorogenic acid, chrysoeriol, derulic acid, eriodictyol, eugenol, 4-terpinol, gallic acid, gamma-terpinene, isochlorogenic acid, isoeugenol, isothymonin, kaemferol, labiatic acid, lauric acid, linalyl acetate, luteolin, methionine, myrcene, myristic acid, naringenin, rosmarinic acid, selenium, tannin, thymol, tryptophan, ursolic acid, vanillic acid.

This is what you ingest when you eat food flavored with thyme. Some of these chemicals are broken down by your digestion, but others go on to do various as-yet-undetermined things to your body: turning some gene's expression on or off, perhaps, or intercepting a free radical before it disturbs a strand of DNA deep in some cell. It would be great to know how this all works, but in the meantime we can enjoy thyme in the knowledge that it probably doesn't do any harm (since people have been eating it forever) and that it might actually do some good (since people have been eating it forever), and even if it does nothing at all, we like the way it tastes.

It's important also to remind ourselves that what reductive science can manage to perceive well enough to isolate and study is subject to almost continual change, and that we have a tendency to assume that what we *can* see is the important thing to look at. The vast attention paid to cholesterol since the 1950s is largely the result of the fact that for a long time cholesterol was the only factor linked to heart disease that we had the tools to measure. (This is sometimes called parking-lot science, after the legendary fellow who loses his keys in a parking lot and goes looking for them under the streetlight — not because that's where he lost them but because that's where it's easiest to see.) When we learned how to measure different types of cholesterol, and then triglycerides and C-reactive protein, those became the important components to study. There will no doubt be other factors as yet unidentified. It's an old story: When Prout and Liebig nailed down the macronutrients, scientists figured that they now understood the nature of food and what the body needed from it. Then when the vitamins were isolated a few decades later, scientists thought, okay, now we *really* understand food and what the body needs for its health; and today it's the polyphenols and carotenoids that seem to have completed the picture. But who knows what else is going on deep in the soul of a carrot?

The good news is that, to the carrot eater, it doesn't matter. That's the great thing about eating foods as compared with nutrients: You don't need to fathom a carrot's complexity in order to reap its benefits.

The mystery of the antioxidants points up the danger in taking a nutrient out of the context of food; scientists make a second, related error when they attempt to study the food out of the context of the diet. We eat foods in combinations and in orders that can affect how they're metabolized. The carbohydrates in a bagel will be absorbed more slowly if the bagel is spread with peanut butter; the fiber, fat, and protein in the peanut butter cushion the insulin response, thereby blunting the impact of the carbohydrates. (This is why eating dessert at the end of the meal rather than the beginning is probably a good idea.) Drink coffee with your steak, and your body won't be able to fully absorb the iron in the meat. The olive oil with which I eat tomatoes makes the lycopene they contain more available to my body. Some of those compounds in the sprig of thyme may affect my digestion of the dish I add it to, helping to break down one compound or stimulate production of an enzyme needed to detoxify another. We have barely begun to understand the relationships among foods in a cuisine.

But we do understand some of the simplest relationships among foods, like the zero-sum relationship: If you eat a lot of one thing, you're probably not eating a lot of something else. This fact alone may have helped lead the diet-heart researchers astray. Like most of us, they assumed that a bad outcome like heart disease must have a bad cause, like saturated fat or cholesterol, so they focused their investigative energies on how these bad nutrients might cause disease rather than on how the absence of something else, like plant foods or fish, might figure in the etiology of the disease. Nutrition science has usually put more of its energies into the idea that the problems it studies are the result of too much of a bad thing instead of too little of a good thing. Is this good science or nutritionist prejudice? The epidemiologist John Powles has suggested this predilection is little more than a Puritan bias: *Bad things happen to people who eat bad things.*

But what people *don't* eat may matter as

much as what they do. This fact could explain why populations that eat diets containing lots of animal food generally have higher rates of coronary heart disease and cancer than those that don't. But nutritionism encouraged researchers to look beyond the possibly culpable food itself — meat — to the culpable nutrient in the meat, which scientists have long assumed to be the saturated fat. So they are baffled indeed when large dietary trials like the Women's Health Initiative and the Nurses' Health Study fail to find evidence that reducing fat intake significantly reduces the incidence of heart disease or cancer.

Of course thanks to the low-fat-diet fad (inspired by the same reductionist hypothesis about fat), it is entirely possible to slash your intake of saturated fat without greatly reducing your consumption of animal protein: Just drink the low-fat milk, buy the low-fat cheese, and order the chicken breast or the turkey bacon instead of the burger. So did the big dietary trials exonerate meat or just fat? Unfortunately, the focus on nutrients didn't tell us much about *foods*. Perhaps the culprit nutrient in meat and dairy is the animal protein itself, as some researchers hypothesize. (The Cornell nutritionist T. Colin Campbell argues as

97

much in his recent book, *The China Study.*)
Others think it could be the particular kind
of iron in red meat (called heme iron) or
the nitrosamines produced when meat is
cooked. Perhaps it is the steroid growth
hormones typically present in the milk and
meat; these hormones (which occur naturally in meat and milk but are often aug-
mented in industrial production) are known
to promote certain kinds of cancer.

Or, as I mentioned, the problem with a
meat-heavy diet might not even be the meat
itself but the plants that all that meat has
pushed off the plate. We just don't know.
But eaters worried about their health
needn't wait for science to settle this question before deciding that it might be wise to
eat more plants and less meat. This of
course is precisely what the McGovern
committee was trying to tell us.

The zero-sum fallacy of nutrition science
poses another obstacle to nailing down the
effect of a single nutrient. As Gary Taubes
points out, it's difficult to design a dietary
trial of something like saturated fat because
as soon as you remove it from the trial diet,
either you have dramatically reduced the
calories in that diet or you have replaced
the saturated fat with something else: other
fats (but which ones?), or carbohydrates

(but what kind?), or protein. Whatever you do, you've introduced a second variable into the experiment, so you will not be able to attribute any observed effect strictly to the absence of saturated fat. It could just as easily be due to the reduction in calories or the addition of carbohydrates or polyunsaturated fats. For every diet hypothesis you test, you can construct an alternative hypothesis based on the presence or absence of the substitute nutrient. It gets messy.

And then there is the placebo effect, which has always bedeviled nutrition research. About a third of Americans are what researchers call responders — people who will respond to a treatment or intervention regardless of whether they've actually received it. When testing a drug you can correct for this by using a placebo in your trial, but how do you correct for the placebo effect in the case of a dietary trial? You can't: Low-fat foods seldom taste like the real thing, and no person is ever going to confuse a meat entrée for a vegetarian substitute.

Marion Nestle also cautions against taking the diet out of the context of the lifestyle, a particular hazard when comparing the diets of different populations. The Mediterranean diet is widely believed to be one of the most healthful traditional diets, yet much of what we know about it is based on studies of people living in the 1950s on the island of Crete — people who in many respects led lives very different from our own. Yes, they ate lots of olive oil and more fish than meat. But they also did more physical labor. As followers of the Greek Orthodox church, they fasted frequently. They ate lots of wild greens — weeds. And, perhaps most significant, they ate far fewer total calories than we do. Similarly, much of what we know about the health benefits of a vegetarian diet is based on studies of Seventh-Day Adventists, who muddy the nutritional picture by abstaining from alcohol and tobacco as well as meat. These extraneous but unavoidable factors are called, aptly, confounders.

One last example: People who take supplements are healthier than the population at large, yet their health probably has nothing whatsoever to do with the supplements they take — most of which recent studies have suggested are worthless. Supplement takers tend to be better educated, more affluent people who, almost by definition, take a greater than usual interest in personal health — confounders that probably account for their superior health.

But if confounding factors of lifestyle

bedevil epidemiological comparisons of different populations, the supposedly more rigorous studies of large American populations suffer from their own arguably even more disabling flaws. In ascending order of supposed reliability, nutrition researchers have three main methods for studying the impact of diet on health: the case-control study, the cohort study, and the intervention trial. All three are seriously flawed in different ways.

In the case-control study, researchers attempt to determine the diet of a subject who has been diagnosed with a chronic disease in order to uncover its cause. One problem is that when people get sick they may change the way they eat, so the diet they report may not be the diet responsible for their illness. Another problem is that these patients will typically report eating large amounts of whatever the evil nutrient of the moment is. These people read the newspaper too; it's only natural to search for the causes of one's misfortune and, perhaps, to link one's illness to one's behavior. One of the more pernicious aspects of nutritionism is that it encourages us to blame our health problems on lifestyle choices, implying that the individual bears ultimate responsibility for whatever illnesses befall him. It's worth keeping in mind that a far more powerful predictor of heart disease than either diet or exercise is social class.

Long-term observational studies of cohort groups such as the Nurses' Health Study represent a big step up in reliability from the case-control study. For one thing, the studies are prospective rather than retrospective: They begin tracking subjects before they become ill. The Nurses' Study, which has collected data on the eating habits and health outcomes of more than one hundred thousand women over several decades (at a cost of more than one hundred million dollars), is considered the best study of its kind, yet it too has limitations. One is its reliance on food-frequency questionnaires (about which more in a moment). Another is the population of nurses it has chosen to study. Critics (notably Colin Campbell) point out that the sample is relatively uniform and is even more carnivorous than the U.S. population as a whole. Pretty much everyone in the group eats a Western diet. This means that when researchers divide the subject population into groups (typically fifths) to study the impact of, say, a low-fat diet, the quintile eating the lowest-fat diet is not all that low — or so dramatically different from the quintile consuming the highest-fat diet. "Virtually this entire cohort of nurses is consuming a high-risk diet," according to Campbell. That might explain why the Nurses' Study has failed to detect significant benefits for many of the dietary interventions it's looked at. In a subject population that is eating a fairly standard Western diet, as this one is, you're never going to capture the effects, good or bad, of more radically different ways of eating. (In his book, Campbell reports Walter Willett's personal response to this criticism: "You may be right, Colin, but people don't want to go there.")

The so-called gold standard in nutrition research is the large-scale intervention study. In these studies, of which the Women's Health Initiative is the biggest and best known, a large population is divided into two groups. The intervention group changes its diet in some prescribed way while the control group (one hopes) does not. The two groups are then tracked over many years to learn whether the intervention affects relative rates of chronic disease. In the case of the Women's Health Initiative study of dietary fat, a $415 million undertaking sponsored by the National Institutes of Health, the eating habits and health outcomes of nearly forty-nine thousand women (aged fifty to seventy-nine) were tracked for eight years to assess the impact of a low-fat diet on a woman's risk of breast and colorectal cancer and cardiovascular disease. Forty percent of the women were told to reduce their consumption of fat to 20 percent of total calories. When the results were announced in 2006, it made front-page news (*The New York Times* headline said LOW-FAT DIET DOES NOT CUT HEALTH RISKS, STUDY FINDS) and the cloud of nutritional confusion beneath which Americans endeavor to eat darkened further.

Even a cursory examination of the study's methods makes you wonder what, if anything, it proved, either about dietary fat or meat eating. You could argue that, like the Nurses' Healthy Study, all any such trials prove is that changing one component in the diet at a time, and not by much, does not confer a significant health benefit. But perhaps the strongest conclusion that can be drawn from an analysis of the Women's Health Initiative is about the inherent limitations of this kind of nutrient-by-nutrient nutrition research.

Even the beginning student of nutritionism will immediately spot several flaws: The focus was on dietary fat rather than on any particular food, such as meat or dairy. So women could reach their goal simply by switching to lower-fat animal products. Also, no distinctions were made between different types of fat: Women getting their allowable portion of fat from olive oil or fish were lumped together with women getting their fat from low-fat cheese or chicken breasts or margarine. Why? Because when the study was designed sixteen years ago, the whole notion of "good fats" was not yet on the mainstream scientific scope. Scientists study what scientists can see.

Another problem with the trial was that the low-fat group failed to hit the target of reducing their fat intake to 20 percent of total calories. The best they could manage was 24 percent in the first year, but by the end of the study they'd drifted back to 29 percent, only a few percentage points lower than the control group's fat intake. Which was itself drifting downward as the women allowed to eat as much fat as they wanted presumably read the newspapers and the food product labels and absorbed the culture's enthusiasm for all things low fat. (This corruption of a control group by popular dietary advice is called the treatment effect.) So it's hardly surprising that the health outcomes of the two groups would not greatly differ — by the end, they might have been consuming pretty much the same diet.

I say "might have been" because we actually have little idea what these women were really eating. Like most people asked about their diet, they lied about it — which brings us to what is perhaps the single biggest problem in doing nutrition science. Even the scientists who conduct this sort of research conduct it in the knowledge that people underestimate (let's be generous) their food intake all the time. They have even developed scientific figures for the magnitude of the error. "Validation studies" of dietary trials like the Women's Health Initiative or the Nurses' Study, which rely on "food-frequency questionnaires" filled out by subjects several times a year, indicate that people on average eat between a fifth and a third more than they say they do on questionnaires.* How do the researchers

*In fact, the magnitude of the error could be much greater, judging by the huge disparity between the total number of food calories produced every day for each American (3,900) and the average number of those calories Americans own up to chomping each day: 2,000. Waste can account for some of this disparity, but not nearly all of it.

know that? By comparing what people report on their food-frequency question-naires with interviews about their dietary intake over the previous twenty-four hours, thought to be somewhat more reliable. Somewhat. Because as you might expect, these "twenty-four-hour recall" data have their own accuracy problems: How typical of your overall diet is what you ate during any single twenty-four-hour period?

To try to fill out the food-frequency questionnaire used by the Women's Health Initiative, as I recently did, is to realize just how shaky the data on which all such dietary studies rely really are. The survey, which takes about forty-five minutes to complete, starts off with some relatively easy questions. "Did you eat chicken or turkey during the last three months?" Having answered yes, I then was asked, "When you ate chicken or turkey, how often did you eat the skin?" And, "Did you usually choose light meat, dark meat, both?" But the survey soon became harder, as when it asked me to think back over the past three months to recall whether when I ate okra, squash, or yams were they fried, and if so, were they fried in stick margarine, tub margarine, butter, shortening (in which category they inexplicably lumped together hydrogenated vegetable oil and lard), olive or canola oil, or nonstick spray? I would hope they'd take my answers with a grain of salt because I honestly didn't remember and in the case of any okra eaten in a restaurant, even a hypnotist or CIA interrogator could not extract from me what sort of fat it was fried in. Now that we spend half of our food dollars on meals prepared outside of the home, how can respondents possibly know what type of fats they're consuming?

Matters got even sketchier in the second section of the survey, when I was asked to specify how many times in the last three months I'd eaten a half-cup serving of broccoli, among a dizzying array of other fruits and vegetables I was asked to tally for the dietary quarter. I'm not sure Marcel Proust himself could recall his dietary intake over the last ninety days with the sort of precision demanded by the FFQ.

When you get to the meat section, the portion sizes specified haven't been seen in America since the Hoover administration. If a four-ounce portion of steak is considered "medium," was I really going to admit that the steak I enjoyed on an unrecallable number of occasions during the past three months was probably the equivalent of two or three (or in the case of a steak house steak, no fewer than *four*) of these portions? I think not. In fact, most of the "medium serving sizes" to which I was asked to compare my own consumption made me feel like such a pig that I badly wanted to shave a few ounces here, a few there. (I mean, I wasn't under oath or anything.)

These are the sort of data on which the largest questions of diet and health are being decided today. "The most intellectually demanding challenge in the field of nutrition," as Marion Nestle writes in *Food Politics,* "is to determine dietary intake." The uncomfortable fact is that the entire field of nutritional science rests on a foundation of ignorance and lies about the most basic question of nutrition: What are people eating? Over lunch, I asked Nestle if I was perhaps being too harsh. She smiled.

"To really know what a person is eating you'd have to have a second invisible person following them around, taking photographs, looking at ingredients, and consulting accurate food composition tables, which we don't have." When you report on an FFQ that you ate a carrot, the tabulator consults a U.S. Department of Agriculture database to determine exactly how much calcium or beta-carotene that carrot contained. But because all carrots are not created equal, their nutrient content varying with everything from the variety planted and type of soil it was planted in to the agriculture system used (organic? conventional?) and the carrot's freshness, these tables suffer from their own inaccuracies.

I was beginning to realize just how much suspension of disbelief it takes to be a nutrition scientist.

"It's impossible," Nestle continued. "Are people unconsciously underestimating consumption of things they think the researcher thinks are bad or overestimating consumption of things they think the researcher thinks are good? We don't know. Probably both. The issue of reporting is extraordinarily serious. We have to ask, How accurate are the data?"

It's not as though the epidemiologists who develop and deploy FFQs are unaware of their limitations. Some of them, like Walter Willett, strive heroically to repair the faulty data, developing "energy adjustment" factors to correct for the fact that the calories reported on surveys are invariably wrong and complicated "measurement error" algorithms to fix the errors in the twenty-four-hour recall surveys used to fix the errors in the FFQ.

I tracked down Gladys Block, the prominent epidemiologist who developed the FFQ on which the Women's Health Initiative based its own questionnaire. We met for coffee in Berkeley, where she is a professor in the School of Public Health. Nearing retirement, Block is unusually thoughtful about the limits of her field and disarmingly candid. "It's a mess," she said, speaking not of the FFQ itself but of the various formulae and algorithms being used to correct errors in the data. "Because if the energy [i.e., the reported calorie consumption] is off, then the nutrients are off too. So if you're going to correct for calories, do you then also correct for . . ." She paused and then sighed. "No, it's a mess."

Block thinks the problem with nutrition science, which she feels "has led us astray," is not the FFQ itself but mis- and overinterpretation of the data derived from the FFQ, a tool for which she makes realistic but strikingly modest claims: "The real purpose of the FFQ is to rank people" on their relative consumption of, say, fruits and vegetables or total calories. "If someone reports consuming five hundred calories a day, that's not true, obviously, but you *can* say they're probably at the low end of the spectrum. People overworry about accuracy."

This was not the sort of thing I expected to hear from an epidemiologist. But then neither was this: "I don't believe anything I read in nutritional epidemiology anymore. I'm so skeptical at this point."

TEN:
NUTRITIONISM'S CHILDREN

So where does this leave us eaters? More confused about how to eat than any people in history, would be my strictly unscientific conclusion. Actually, there *is* some science, admittedly a little soft, which has captured a bit of the confusion that the supposedly harder science of nutrition has sown in the American mind. Paul Rozin is a psychologist at the University of Pennsylvania who has dreamed up some of the more imaginative survey questions ever asked of American eaters; the answers he's collected offer a pretty good index to our current befuddlement and anxiety about eating. He has found, for example, that half of us believe high-calorie foods eaten in small amounts contain more calories than low-calorie foods eaten in much larger amounts. And that a third of us believe that a diet absolutely free of fat — a nutrient, lest you forget, essential to our survival — would be better for us than a diet containing even just "a pinch" of it. In one experiment, he showed the words "chocolate cake" to a group of Americans and recorded their word associations. "Guilt" was the top response. If that strikes you as unexceptional, consider the response of the French eaters to the same prompt: "celebration." (Oh, yeah.) I think of Rozin as a kind of psychoanalyst of nutritionism.

A few years ago, Rozin presented a group of Americans with the following scenario: "Assume you are alone on a desert island for one year and you can have water and one other food. Pick the food that you think would be best for your health."

The choices were corn, alfalfa sprouts, hot dogs, spinach, peaches, bananas, and milk chocolate. The most popular choice was bananas (42 percent), followed by spinach (27 percent), corn (12 percent), alfalfa sprouts (7 percent), peaches (5 percent), hot dogs (4 percent), and milk chocolate (3 percent). Only 7 percent of the participants chose one of the two foods that would in fact best support survival: hot dogs and milk chocolate.

Evidently some of the wreckage of the lipid hypothesis has washed up on Rozin's desert island.

"Fat," he writes, "seems to have assumed,

even at low levels, the role of a toxin" in our dietary imaginations. I wonder why. As Rozin points out, "Worrying so much about food can't be very good for your health." Indeed. Orthorexia nervosa is an eating disorder not yet recognized by the DSM-IV, but some psychologists have recently suggested that it's time it was. They're seeing more and more patients suffering from "an unhealthy obsession with healthy eating."

So this is what putting science, and scientism, in charge of the American diet has gotten us: anxiety and confusion about even the most basic questions of food and health, and a steadily diminishing ability to enjoy one of the great pleasures of life without guilt or neurosis.

But while nutritionism has its roots in a scientific approach to food, it's important to remember that it is not a science but an ideology, and that the food industry, journalism, and government bear just as much responsibility for its conquest of our minds and diets. All three helped to amplify the signal of nutritionism: journalism by uncritically reporting the latest dietary studies on its front pages; the food industry by marketing dubious foodlike products on the basis of tenuous health claims; and the government by taking it upon itself to issue official dietary advice based on sketchy science in the first place and corrupted by political pressure in the second. The novel food products the industry designed according to the latest nutritionist specs certainly helped push real food off our plates. But the industry's influence would not be nearly so great had the ideology of nutritionism not already undermined the influence of tradition and habit and common sense — and the transmitter of all those values, mom — on our eating.

Now, all this *might* be tolerable if eating by the light of nutritionism made us, if not happier, then at least healthier. That it has failed to do. Thirty years of nutritional advice have left us fatter, sicker, and more poorly nourished. Which is why we find ourselves in the predicament we do: in need of a whole new way to think about eating.

■ ■ ■ ■

II

THE WESTERN DIET AND THE DISEASES OF CIVILIZATION

■ ■ ■ ■

ONE:
THE ABORIGINE IN
ALL OF US

In the summer of 1982, a group of ten middle-aged, overweight, and diabetic Aborigines living in settlements near the town of Derby, Western Australia, agreed to participate in an experiment to see if temporarily reversing the process of westernization they had undergone might also reverse their health problems. Since leaving the bush some years before, all ten had developed type 2 diabetes; they also showed signs of insulin resistance (when the body's cells lose their sensitivity to insulin) and elevated levels of triglycerides in the blood — a risk factor for heart disease. "Metabolic syndrome," or "syndrome X," is the medical term for the complex of health problems these Aborigines had developed: Large amounts of refined carbohydrates in the diet combined with a sedentary lifestyle had disordered the intricate (and still imperfectly understood) system by which the insulin hormone regulates the metabolism of carbo-hydrates and fats in the body. Metabolic syndrome has been implicated not only in the development of type 2 diabetes, but also in obesity, hypertension, heart disease, and possibly certain cancers. Some researchers believe that metabolic syndrome may be at the root of many of the "diseases of civiliza-tion" that typically follow a native popula-tion's adoption of a Western lifestyle and the nutrition transition that typically entails.

The ten Aborigines returned to their traditional homeland, an isolated region of northwest Australia more than a day's drive by off-road vehicle from the nearest town. From the moment they left civilization, the men and women in the group had no ac-cess to store food or beverages; the idea was for them to rely exclusively on foods they hunted and gathered themselves. (Even while living in town, they still occasionally hunted traditional foods and so had pre-served the knowledge of how to do so.) Kerin O'Dea, the nutrition researcher who designed the experiment, accompanied the group to monitor and record its dietary intake and keep tabs on the members' health.

The Aborigines divided their seven-week stay in the bush between a coastal and an inland location. While on the coast, their diet consisted mainly of seafood, supplemented by birds, kangaroo, and witchetty grubs, the fatty larvae of a local insect. Hoping to find more plant foods, the group moved inland after two weeks, settling at a riverside location. Here, in addition to freshwater fish and shellfish, the diet expanded to include turtle, crocodile, birds, kangaroo, yams, figs, and bush honey. The contrast between this hunter-gatherer fare and their previous diet was stark: O'Dea reports that prior to the experiment "the main dietary components in the urban setting were flour, sugar, rice, carbonated drinks, alcoholic beverages (beer and port), powdered milk, cheap fatty meat, potatoes, onions, and variable contributions of other fresh fruits and vegetables" — the local version of the Western diet.

After seven weeks in the bush, O'Dea drew blood from the Aborigines and found striking improvements in virtually every measure of their health. All had lost weight (an average of 17.9 pounds) and seen their blood pressure drop. Their triglyceride levels had fallen into the normal range. The proportion of omega-3 fatty acids in their tissues had increased dramatically. "In summary," O'Dea concluded, "all of the metabolic abnormalities of type II diabetes were either greatly improved (glucose tolerance, insulin response to glucose) or completely normalized (plasma lipids) in a group of diabetic Aborigines by a relatively short (seven week) reversion to traditional hunter-gatherer lifestyle."

O'Dea does not report what happened next, whether the Aborigines elected to remain in the bush or return to civilization, but it's safe to assume that if they did return to their Western lifestyles, their health problems returned too. We have known for a century now that there is a complex of so-called Western diseases — including obesity, diabetes, cardiovascular disease, hypertension, and a specific set of diet-related cancers — that begin almost invariably to appear soon after a people abandons its traditional diet and way of life. What we did not know before O'Dea took her Aborigines back to the bush (and since she did, a series of comparable experiments have produced similar results in Native Americans and native Hawaiians) was that some of the most deleterious effects of the Western diet could be so quickly reversed. It appears that, at least to an extent, we can rewind the tape of the nutrition transition and undo some of its damage. The implications for our own health are potentially significant.[*]

The genius of Kerin O'Dea's experiment

[*]According to Walter C. Willett, only 3.1 percent of the Nurses' Health Study population could be described as following a "low risk" diet and lifestyle, which he defines as follows: nonsmoker, body-mass index (BMI) below 25 (the threshold for overweight), thirty minutes of exercise a day, and a diet characterized by low intake of trans fat; high ratio of polyunsaturated to saturated fats; high whole-grain intake; two servings of fish a week; recommended daily allowance of folic acid and at least five grams of alcohol a day. Based on fourteen years of follow-up, Willett and his colleagues calculated that, had the entire cohort adopted these behaviors, 80 percent of coronary heart disease; 90 percent of type 2 diabetes, and more than 70 percent of colon cancer cases could have been avoided. This analysis suggests that the worst effects of the Western diet can be avoided or reversed without leaving civilization. Or, as Willett writes, "the potential for disease prevention by modest dietary and lifestyle changes that are readily compatible with life in the 21st century is enormous." From Walter C. Willet, "The Pursuit of Optimal Diets: A Progress Report" in Jim Kaput, and Raymond L. Rodriguez, *Nutritional Genomics: Discovering the Path to Personalized Nutrition* (New York: John Wiley & Sons, 2006).

123

was its simplicity — and her refusal to let herself be drawn into the scientific labyrinth of nutritionism. She did not attempt to pick out from the complexity of the diet (either before or after the experiment) which one nutrient might explain the results — whether it was the low-fat diet, or the absence of refined carbohydrates, or the reduction in total calories that was responsible for the improvement in the group's health. Her focus instead was on larger dietary patterns, and while this approach has its limitations (we can't extract from such a study precisely which component of the Western diet we need to adjust in order to blunt its worst effects), it has the great virtue of escaping the welter of conflicting theories about specific nutrients and returning our attention to more fundamental questions about the links between diet and health.

Like this one: To what extent are we all Aborigines? When you consider that two thirds of Americans are overweight or obese, that fully a quarter of us have metabolic syndrome, that fifty-four million have pre-diabetes, and that the incidence of type 2 diabetes has risen 5 percent annually since 1990, going from 4 percent to 7.7 percent of the adult population (that's more than twenty million Americans), the question is not nearly as silly as it sounds.

Two:
The Elephant in the Room

In the end, even the biggest, most ambitious, and widely reported studies of diet and health — the Nurses' Health Study, the Women's Health Initiative, and nearly all the others — leave undisturbed the main features of the Western diet: lots of processed foods and meat, lots of added fat and sugar, lots of everything except fruits, vegetables, and whole grains. In keeping with the nutritionism paradigm and the limits of reductionist science, most nutrition researchers fiddle with single nutrients as best they can, but the populations they recruit and study are typical American eaters doing what typical American eaters do: trying to eat a little less of this nutrient, a little more of that one, depending on the latest thinking. But the overall dietary pattern is treated as a more or less unalterable given. Which is why it probably should not surprise us that the findings of such research should be so modest, equivocal, and confusing.

But what about the elephant in the room

— this pattern of eating that we call the Western diet? In the midst of our deepening confusion about nutrition, it might be useful to step back and gaze upon it — review what we *do* know about the Western diet and its effects on our health. What we know is that people who eat the way we do in the West today suffer substantially higher rates of cancer, cardiovascular diseases, diabetes, and obesity than people eating any number of different traditional diets. We also know that when people come to the West and adopt our way of eating, these diseases soon follow, and often, as in the case of the Aborigines and other native populations, in a particularly virulent form.

The outlines of this story — the story of the so-called Western diseases and their link to the Western diet — we first learned in the early decades of the twentieth century. That was when a handful of dauntless European and American medical professionals working with a wide variety of native populations around the world began noticing the almost complete absence of the chronic diseases that had recently become commonplace in the West. Albert Schweitzer and Denis P. Burkitt in Africa, Robert Mc-Carrison in India, Samuel Hutton among the Eskimos in Labrador, the anthropologist Aleš Hrdlička among Native Americans, and the dentist Weston A. Price among a dozen different groups all over the world (including Peruvian Indians, Australian Aborigines, and Swiss mountaineers) sent back much the same news. They compiled lists, many of which appeared in medical journals, of the common diseases they'd been hard pressed to find in the native populations they had treated or studied: little to no heart disease, diabetes, cancer, obesity, hypertension, or stroke; no appendicitis, diverticulitis, malformed dental arches, or tooth decay; no varicose veins, ulcers, or hemorrhoids. These disorders suddenly appeared to these researchers under a striking new light, as suggested by the name given to them by the British doctor Denis Burkitt, who worked in Africa during World War II: He proposed that we call them Western diseases. The implication was that these very different sorts of diseases were somehow linked and might even have a common cause.

Several of these researchers were on hand to witness the arrival of the Western diseases in isolated populations, typically, as Albert Schweitzer wrote, among "natives living more and more after the manner of the whites." Some noted that the Western diseases followed closely on the heels of the arrival of Western foods, particularly refined flour and sugar and other kinds of "store food." They observed too that when one Western disease arrived on the scene, so did most of the others, and often in the same order: obesity followed by type 2 diabetes followed by hypertension and stroke followed by heart disease.

In the years before World War II the medical world entertained a lively conversation on the subject of the Western diseases and what their rise might say about our increasingly industrialized way of life. The concept's pioneers believed there were novelties in the modern diet to which native populations were poorly adapted, though they did not necessarily agree on exactly which novelty might be the culprit. Burkitt, for example, believed it was the lack of fiber in the modern diet while McCarrison, a British army doctor, focused on refined carbohydrates while still others blamed meat eating and saturated fat or, in Price's case, the advent of processed food and industrially grown crops deficient in vitamins and minerals.

Not everyone, though, bought into the idea that chronic disease was a by-product of Western lifestyles and, in particular, that the industrialization of our food was taking a toll on our health. One objection to the theory was genetic: Different races were apt to be susceptible to different diseases went the argument; white people were disposed to heart attacks, brown people to things like leprosy. Yet as Burkitt and others pointed out, blacks living in America suffered from the same chronic diseases as whites living there. Simply by moving to places like America, immigrants from nations with low rates of chronic disease seemed to quickly acquire them.

The other objection to the concept of Western diseases, one you sometimes still hear, was demographic. The reason we see so much chronic disease in the West is because these are illnesses that appear relatively late in life, and with the conquest of infectious disease early in the twentieth century, we're simply living long enough to get them. In this view, chronic disease is the inevitable price of a long life. But while it is true that our life expectancy has improved dramatically since 1900 (rising in the United States from forty-nine to seventy-seven years), most of that gain is attributed to the fact that more of us are surviving infancy and childhood; the life expectancy of a sixty-five-year-old in 1900 was only about six years less than that of a sixty-five-year-old living today.* When you adjust for age, rates of chronic diseases like cancer and type 2 diabetes are considerably higher today than they were in 1900. That is, the chances that a sixty- or seventy-year-old suffers from cancer or type 2 diabetes are far greater today than they were a century ago. (The same may well be true of heart disease, but because heart disease statistics from 1900 are so sketchy, we can't say for sure.)

Cancer and heart disease and so many of the other Western diseases are by now such an accepted part of modern life that it's hard for us to believe this wasn't always or even necessarily the case. These days most of us think of chronic diseases as being a

*It may be that the explosion of chronic diseases during the twentieth century is now taking a toll on American life expectancy. In 2007, the *CIA World Factbook* ranked the United States forty-fifth for life expectancy at birth, below countries like Israel, Jordan, Bosnia, and Bermuda. Future gains in life expectancy depend largely on how much we can extend life among the elderly — exceedingly difficult, when you consider that the incidence of diabetes in people over seventy-five is projected to increase 336 percent during the first half of this century.

little like the weather — one of life's givens — and so count ourselves lucky that, compared to the weather, the diseases at least are more amenable to intervention by modern medicine. We think of them strictly in medical rather than historical, much less evolutionary, terms. But during the decades before World War II, when the industrialization of so many aspects of our lives was still fairly fresh, the price of "progress," especially to our health, seemed more obvious to many people and therefore more open to question.

One of the most intrepid questioners of the prewar period was Weston A. Price, a Canadian-born dentist, of all things, who became preoccupied with one of those glaring questions we can't even see anymore. Much like heart disease, chronic problems of the teeth are by now part of the furniture of modern life. But if you stop to think about it, it *is* odd that everyone should need a dentist and that so many of us should need braces, root canals, extractions of wisdom teeth, and all the other routine procedures of modern mouth maintenance. Could the need for so much remedial work on a body part crucially involved in an activity as critical to our survival as eating reflect a design defect in the human body, some

131

sort of oversight of natural selection? This seems unlikely. Weston Price, who was born in 1870 in a farming community south of Ottawa and built a dental practice in Cleveland, Ohio, had personally witnessed the rapid increase in dental problems beginning around the turn of the last century and was convinced that the cause could be found in the modern diet. (He wasn't the only one: In the 1930s an argument raged in medical circles as to whether hygiene or nutrition was the key to understanding and treating tooth decay. A public debate on that very question in Manhattan in 1934 attracted an overflow audience of thousands. That hygiene ultimately won the day had as much to do with the needs of the dental profession as it did with good science; the problem of personal hygiene was easier, and far more profitable, to address than that of the diet and entire food system.)

In the 1930s, Price closed down his dental practice so he could devote all his energies to solving the mystery of the Western diet. He went looking for what he called control groups — isolated populations that had not yet been exposed to modern foods. He found them in the mountains of Switzerland and Peru, the lowlands of Africa, the bush of Australia, the outer islands of the Hebrides, the Everglades of Florida, the coast of Alaska, the islands of Melanesia and the Torres Strait, and the jungles of New Guinea and New Zealand, among other places. Price made some remarkable discoveries, which he wrote up in articles for medical journals (with titles like "New Light on Modern Physical Degeneration from Field Studies Among Primitive Races") and ultimately summarized in his 510-page tome, *Nutrition and Physical Degeneration,* published in 1939.

Although his research was taken seriously during his lifetime, Weston Price has been all but written out of the history of twentieth-century science. The single best account I could find of his life and work is an unpublished master's thesis by Martin Renner, a graduate student in history at UC Santa Cruz.* This neglect might owe to the fact that Price was a dentist, and more of an amateur scientist in the nineteenth-century mode than a professional medical researcher. It might also be because he could sometimes come across as a bit of a crackpot — one of his articles was titled

*"Modern Civilization, Nutritional Dark Age: Weston A. Price's Ecological Critique of the Industrial Food System," 2005.

"Dentistry and Race Destiny." His discussions of "primitive races" are off-putting to say the least, though he ended up a harsh critic of "modern civilization," convinced his primitives had more to teach us than the other way around. He was also something of a monomaniac on the subject of diet, certain that poor nutrition could explain not just tooth decay and heart disease but just about everything else that bedeviled humankind, including juvenile delinquency, the collapse of civilizations, and war.

Still, the data he painstakingly gathered from his control groups, and the lines of connection he was able to trace, not only between diet and health but also between the way a people produces food and that food's nutritional quality, remain valuable today. Indeed, his research is even more valuable today than in 1939, because most of the groups he studied have long since vanished or adopted more Western ways of eating. If you want to study the Western diet today, control groups are few and far between. (You can of course create them, as Kerin O'Dea did in Australia.) Price's work also points the way toward a protoecological understanding of food that will be useful as we try to escape the traps of nutritionism.

So what did Price learn? First, that isolated populations eating a wide variety of traditional diets had no need of dentists whatsoever. (Well, *almost* no need of dentists: The "sturdy mountaineers" of Switzerland, who never met a toothbrush, had teeth covered in a greenish slime — but underneath that Price found perfectly formed teeth virtually free of decay.) Wherever he found an isolated primitive race that had not yet encountered the "displacing foods of modern commerce" — by which he meant refined flour, sugar, canned and chemically preserved foods, and vegetable oils — he found little or no evidence of "modern degeneration" — by which he meant chronic disease, tooth decay, and malformed dental arches. Either there was something present in the Western diet that led to these problems or there was something absent from it.

Wherever Price went he took pictures of teeth and collected samples of food, which he sent home to Cleveland to be analyzed for macronutrient and vitamin content. He found that his native populations were eating a diet substantially higher in vitamins A and D than that of modern Americans — on average ten times as much. This owed partly to the fact that, as was already understood by the 1930s, the processing of foods typically robs them of nutrients, vitamins especially. Store food is food designed to be stored and transported over long distances, and the surest way to make food more stable and less vulnerable to pests is to remove the nutrients from it. In general, calories are much easier to transport — in the form of refined grain or sugar — than nutrients, which are liable to deteriorate or attract the attention of bacteria, insects, and rodents, all keenly interested in nutrients. (More so, apparently, than we are.) Price concluded that modern civilization had sacrificed much of the quality of its food in the interests of quantity and shelf life.

Price identified no single ideal diet — he found populations that thrived on seafood diets, dairy diets, meat diets, and diets in which fruits, vegetables, and grain predominated. The Masai of Africa consumed virtually no plant foods at all, subsisting on meat, blood, and milk. Seafaring groups in the Hebrides consumed no dairy at all, subsisting on a diet consisting largely of seafood and oats made into porridges and cakes. The Eskimos he interviewed lived on raw fish, game meat, fish roe, and blubber, seldom eating anything remotely green.

Along the Nile near Ethiopia, Price encountered what he judged to be the healthiest populations of all: tribes that subsisted on milk, meat, and blood from pastured cattle as well as animal food from the Nile River. Price found groups that ate diets of wild animal flesh to be generally healthier than the agriculturists who relied on cereals and other plant foods; the agriculturists tended to have somewhat higher levels of tooth decay (though still low by our standards). Price noted that many of the peoples he visited particularly prized organ meats, in which he found high levels of fat-soluble vitamins, minerals, and "activator X," a term of his own invention that is probably vitamin K_2. Almost everywhere he went, he noted the high value people placed on seafood, which even mountain-dwelling groups would go to great lengths to procure, trading with coastal tribes for dried fish eggs and such. But the common denominator of good health, he concluded, was to eat a traditional diet consisting of fresh foods from animals and plants grown on soils that were themselves rich in nutrients.

Price paid special attention to the quality of animal-based foods and its link to what those animals ate. He compared the vitamin content of butter produced from cows grazing on spring grass to that of animals on winter forages; not only were levels of vitamins A and D much higher in the yellower butter of the pastured animals but the health of the people who subsisted on those animals was better too. Price believed the quality of the soil was a key to health, and in 1932, he published a paper titled "New Light on Some Relationships Between Soil Mineral Deficiencies, Low Vitamin Foods, and Some Degenerative Diseases."

In making such connections between the quality of soil and grass and the health of the human eaters at the top of the food chain, Price was advancing a critique of the industrialized agriculture just getting established in the thirties. In this he was not alone: Around the same time, the English agronomist Sir Albert Howard, the philosophical father of the organic farming movement, was also arguing that the industrialization of agriculture — in particular the introduction of synthetic nitrogen fertilizer, which simplified the chemistry of the soil — would eventually take its toll on our health. Howard urged that we regard "the whole problem of health in soil, plant, animal and man as one great subject." When Howard wrote these words, this was still little more than a working hypothesis;

Weston Price had begun to put some empirical foundations beneath it.

Price was inching toward an ecological understanding of diet and health that was well ahead of his time. He understood that, ultimately, eating linked us to the earth and its elements as well as to the energy of the sun. "The dinner we have eaten tonight," he told his audience in a 1928 lecture, "was a part of the sun but a few months ago." Industrial food both obscured these links and attenuated them. In lengthening the food chain so that we could feed great cities from distant soils, we were breaking the "rules of nature" at least twice: by robbing nutrients from the soils the foods had been grown in and then squandering those nutrients by processing the foods. Compared to the native peoples Price studied, many of whom took pains to return nutrients to the local soil on which they absolutely depended, "our modern civilization returns exceedingly little of what it borrows. Vast fleets are busy carrying the limited minerals of far-flung districts to distant markets." Renner documents how Price eventually came to see the problem of diet and health as a problem of ecological dysfunction. By breaking the links among local soils, local foods, and local peoples, the industrial food system disrupted the circular flow of nutrients through the food chain. Whatever the advantages of the new industrial system, it could no longer meet the biochemical requirements of the human body, which, not having had time to adapt, was failing in new ways.

Whether or not you're willing to travel quite that far with Dr. Price, he and all the other early twentieth-century explorers of the pre-Western diet returned to civilization with the same simple and devastating piece of news, one that seems hard to deny: The human animal is adapted to, and apparently can thrive on, an extraordinary range of different diets, but the Western diet, however you define it, does not seem to be one of them.

As it happened, the ecological critique of industrial civilization that Weston Price was advancing in the thirties would not survive World War II. The space for such writing — occupied also by Sir Howard and Lord Northbourne in England and the American agrarians — closed down very shortly after Price published *Nutrition and Physical Degeneration* in 1939. People would soon lose their patience for attacks on "industrial civilization," that being precisely what they were depending on to save them in wartime.

By the time the war ended, that industrial civilization had consolidated its hold and in the process become much more sure of itself. In the years immediately after the war, industrial agriculture (which benefited from the peacetime conversion of munitions to chemical fertilizer and nerve gas research to pesticides) also consolidated its position; there would soon be no other kind. Weston Price and his fellow students of the Western diseases were largely forgotten. No one was much interested in looking back or celebrating the wisdom of primitive groups that were themselves quickly disappearing or being assimilated; even the Aborigines were moving to the city.

As for the Western diseases, they hadn't gone away — indeed, rates of heart disease exploded immediately after the war — but now they became the responsibility of modern medicine and reductionist science. Nutritionism became the accepted set of terms in which to conduct all conversations about diet and health. It wouldn't be until the late 1960s, with the rise of organic agriculture, that searching questions about the industrial food chain would be posed again.

THREE:
THE INDUSTRIALIZATION OF EATING: WHAT WE DO KNOW

I've dwelled on the all-but-forgotten ideas of people like Weston Price and Sir Albert Howard — ecological thinkers about the human food chain — because they point us down a path that might lead the way out of the narrow, and ultimately unhelpful, confines of nutritionism: of thinking about food strictly in terms of its chemical constituents. What we need now, it seems to me, is to create a broader, more ecological — and more cultural — view of food. So let us try.

What would happen if we were to start thinking about food as less of a thing and more of a relationship? In nature, that is of course precisely what eating has always been: relationships among species in systems we call food chains, or food webs, that reach all the way down to the soil. Species co-evolve with the other species that they eat, and very often there develops a relationship of interdependence: *I'll feed you if you spread around my genes.* A gradual process of mutual adaptation transforms something like an apple or a squash into a nutritious and tasty food for an animal. Over time and through trial and error, the plant becomes tastier (and often more conspicuous) in order to gratify the animal's needs and desires, while the animal gradually acquires whatever digestive tools (enzymes, for example) it needs to make optimal use of the plant.

Similarly, the milk of cows did not start out as a nutritious food for humans; in fact, it made them sick until people who lived around cows evolved the ability to digest milk as adults. The gene for the production of a milk-digesting enzyme called lactase used to switch off in humans shortly after weaning until about five thousand years ago, when a mutation that kept the gene switched on appeared and quickly spread through a population of animal herders in north-central Europe. Why? Because the people possessing the new mutation then had access to a terrifically nutritious new food source and as a consequence were able to produce more offspring than the people who lacked it. This development proved much to the advantage of both the milk drinkers and the cows, whose numbers and habitat (and health) greatly improved as a result of this new symbiotic relationship.

Health is, among other things, the product of being in these sorts of relationships in a food chain — a great many such relation- ships in the case of an omnivorous creature like man. It follows that when the health of one part of the food chain is disturbed, it can affect all the other creatures in it. If the soil is sick or in some way deficient, so will be the grasses that grow in that soil and the cattle that eat the grasses and the people who drink the milk from them. This is precisely what Weston Price and Sir Howard had in mind when they sought to connect the seemingly distant realms of soil and hu- man health. Our personal health cannot be divorced from the health of the entire food web.

In many cases, long familiarity between foods and their eaters leads to elaborate systems of communication up and down the food chain so that a creature's senses come to recognize foods as suitable by their taste and smell and color. Very often these signals are "sent" by the foods themselves, which may have their own reasons for wanting to be eaten. Ripeness in fruit is often signaled by a distinctive smell (an appealing scent that can travel over distances), or color (one that stands out from the general green), or taste (typically sweet). Ripeness, which is the moment when the seeds of the plant are ready to go off and germinate, typically coincides with the greatest concentration of nutrients in a fruit, so the interests of the plant (for transportation) align with those of the plant eater (for nutriment). Our bodies, having received these signals and determined this fruit is good to eat, now produce in anticipation precisely the enzymes and acids needed to break it down. Health depends heavily on knowing how to read these biological signals: *This looks ripe; this smells spoiled; that's one slick-looking cow.* This is much easier to do when you have long experience of a food and much harder when a food has been expressly designed to deceive your senses with, say, artificial flavors or synthetic sweeteners. Foods that lie to our senses are one of the most challenging features of the Western diet.

Note that these ecological relationships are, at least in the first instance, between eaters and whole foods, not nutrients or chemicals. Even though the foods in question eventually get broken down in our bodies into simple chemical compounds, as corn is reduced mostly to simple sugars, the qualities of the whole foods are not unimportant. The amount and structure of the fiber in that corn, for example, will determine such things as the speed at which the sugars in it will be released and absorbed, something we've learned is critical to insulin metabolism. The chemist will tell you the starch in corn is on its way to becoming glucose in the blood, but that reductive understanding overlooks the complex and variable process by which that happens. Contrary to the nutrition label, not all carbohydrates are created equal.

Put another way, our bodies have a long-standing and sustainable relationship to corn that they do not have to high-fructose corn syrup. Such a relationship with corn syrup might develop someday (as people evolve superhuman insulin systems to cope with regular floods of pure fructose and glucose[*]), but for now the relationship leads to ill health because our bodies don't know how to handle these biological novelties. In much the same way, human bodies that can cope with chewing coca leaves — a long-standing relationship between native people and the coca plant in parts of South

[*]Glucose is a sugar molecule that is the body's main source of energy; most carbohydrates are broken down to glucose during digestion. Fructose is a different form of sugar, commonly found in fruit. Sucrose, or table sugar, is a disaccharide consisting of a molecule of glucose joined to a molecule of fructose.

America — cannot cope with cocaine or crack, even though the same active ingredients are present in all three. Reductionism as a way of understanding food or drugs may be harmless, even necessary, but reductionism in practice — reducing food or drug plants to their most salient chemical compounds — can lead to problems.

Looking at eating, and food, through this ecological lens opens a whole new perspective on exactly what the Western diet is: a radical and, at least in evolutionary terms, abrupt set of changes over the course of the last 150 years, not just to our foodstuffs but also to our food relationships, all the way from the soil to the meal. The rise of the ideology of nutritionism is itself part of that change. When we think of a species' "environment," we usually think in terms of things like geography, predators and prey, and the weather. But of course one of the most critical components of any creature's environment is the nature of the food available to it and its relationships to the species it eats. Much is at stake when a creature's food environment changes. For us, the first big change came ten thousand years ago with the advent of agriculture. (And it devastated our health, leading to a panoply of deficiencies and infectious diseases that we've only managed to get under control in the last century or so.) The biggest change in our food environment since then? The advent of the modern diet.

To get a better grip on the nature of these changes is to begin to understand how we might alter our relationship to food — for the better, for our health. These changes have been numerous and far reaching, but consider as a start these five fundamental transformations to our foods and ways of eating. All of them can be reversed, if not perhaps so easily in the food system as a whole, certainly in the life and diet of any individual eater, and without, I hasten to add, returning to the bush or taking up hunting and gathering.

1) From Whole Foods to Refined

The case of corn points to one of the key features of the modern diet: a shift toward increasingly refined foods, especially carbohydrates. People have been refining cereal grains since at least the Industrial Revolution, favoring white flour and white rice over brown, even at the price of lost nutrients. Part of the reason was prestige: Because for many years only the wealthy could afford refined grains, they acquired a certain glamour. Refining grains extends their shelf life (precisely because they are less nutritious to the pests that compete with us for their calories) and makes them easier to digest by removing the fiber that ordinarily slows the release of their sugars. Also, the finer that flour is ground, the more surface area is exposed to digestive enzymes, so the quicker the starches turn to glucose. A great deal of modern industrial food can be seen as an extension and intensification of this practice as food processors find ways to deliver glucose — the brain's preferred fuel — ever more swiftly and efficiently. Sometimes this is precisely the point, as when corn is refined into corn syrup; other times, though, it is an unfortunate by-product of processing food for other reasons.

Viewed from this perspective, the history of refining whole foods has been a history of figuring out ways not just to make them more durable and portable, but also how to concentrate their energy and, in a sense, speed them up. This acceleration took a great leap forward with the introduction in Europe around 1870 of rollers (made from iron, steel, or porcelain) for grinding grain. Perhaps more than any other single development, this new technology, which by 1880 had replaced grinding by stone throughout Europe and America, marked the beginning of the industrialization of our food — reducing it to its chemical essence and speeding up its absorption. Refined flour is the first fast food.

Before the roller-milling revolution, wheat was ground between big stone wheels, which could get white flour only so white. That's because while stone grinding removed the bran from the wheat kernel (and therefore the largest portion of the fiber), it couldn't remove the germ, or embryo, which contains volatile oils that are rich in nutrients. The stone wheels merely crushed the germ and released the oil. This had the effect of tinting the flour yellowish gray (the yellow is carotene) and shortening its shelf life, because the oil, once exposed to the air, soon oxidized — turned rancid. That's what people could see and smell, and they didn't like it. What their senses couldn't tell them, however, is that the germ contributed some of the most valuable nutrients to the flour, including much of its protein, folic acid, and other B vitamins; carotenes and other antioxidants; and omega-3 fatty acids, which are especially prone to rancidity.

The advent of rollers that made it possible to remove the germ and then grind the remaining endosperm (the big packet of starch and protein in a seed) exceptionally fine solved the problem of stability and color. Now just about everyone could afford snowy-white flour that could keep on a shelf for many months. No longer did every town need its own mill, because flour could now travel great distances. (Plus it could be ground year-round by large companies in big cities: Heavy stone mills, which typically relied on water power, operated mostly when and where rivers flowed; steam engines could drive the new rollers whenever and wherever.) Thus was one of the main staples of the Western diet cut loose from its moorings in place and time and marketed on the basis of image rather than nutritional value. In this, white flour was a modern industrial food, one of the first.

The problem was that this gorgeous white powder was nutritionally worthless, or nearly so. Much the same was now true for corn flour and white rice, the polishing of which (i.e., the removing of its most nutritious parts) was perfected around the same time. Wherever these refining technologies came into widespread use, devastating epidemics of pellagra and beriberi soon followed. Both are diseases caused by deficiencies in the B vitamins that the germ had contributed to the diet. But the sudden absence from bread of several other micronutrients, as well as omega-3 fatty acids, probably also took its toll on public health, particularly among the urban poor of Europe, many of whom ate little but bread.

In the 1930s, with the discovery of vitamins, scientists figured out what had happened, and millers began fortifying refined grain with B vitamins. This took care of the most obvious deficiency diseases. More recently, scientists recognized that many of us also had a deficiency of folic acid in our diet, and in 1996 public health authorities ordered millers to start adding folic acid to flour as well. But it would take longer still for science to realize that this "Wonder Bread" strategy of supplementation, as one nutritionist has called it, might not solve all the problems caused by the refining of grain. Deficiency diseases are much easier to trace and treat (indeed, medicine's success in curing deficiency diseases is an important source of nutritionism's prestige) than chronic diseases, and it turns out that the practice of refining carbohydrates is implicated in several of these chronic diseases as well — diabetes, heart disease, and certain cancers.

The story of refined grain stands as a parable about the limits of reductionist science when applied to something as complex as food. For years now nutritionists have known that a diet high in whole grains reduces one's risk for diabetes, heart disease, and cancer. (This seems to be true even after you correct for the fact that the kind of people who eat lots of whole grains today probably have lifestyles healthier in other ways as well.) Different nutritionists have given the credit for the benefits of whole grain to different nutrients: the fiber in the bran, the folic acid and other B vitamins in the germ, or the antioxidants or the various minerals. In 2003 the *American Journal of Clinical Nutrition*[*] published an unusually nonreductionist study demonstrating that no one of those nutrients alone can explain the benefits of whole-grain foods: The typical reductive analysis of isolated nutrients could not explain the improved health of the whole-grain eaters.

For the study, University of Minnesota epidemiologists David R. Jacobs and Lyn M. Steffen reviewed the relevant research and found a large body of evidence that a

[*]David R. Jacobs and Lyn M. Steffen, "Nutrients, Foods, and Dietary Patterns as Exposures in Research: A Framework for Food Synergy," *American Journal of Clinical Nutrition*, 2003; 78 (suppl): 508S–13S.

diet rich in whole grains did in fact reduce mortality from all causes. But what was surprising was that even after adjusting for levels of dietary fiber, vitamin E, folic acid, phytic acid, iron, zinc, magnesium, and manganese in the diet (all the good things we know are in whole grains), they found an additional health benefit to eating whole grains that none of the nutrients alone or even together could explain. That is, subjects getting the same amounts of these nutrients from other sources were not as healthy as the whole-grain eaters. "This analysis suggests that something else in the whole grain protects against death." The authors concluded, somewhat vaguely but suggestively, that "the various grains and their parts act synergistically" and suggested that their colleagues begin paying attention to the concept of "food synergy." Here, then, is support for an idea revolutionary by the standards of nutritionism: A whole food might be more than the sum of its nutrient parts.

Suffice it to say, this proposition has not been enthusiastically embraced by the food industry, and probably won't be any time soon. As I write, Coca-Cola is introducing vitamin-fortified sodas, extending the Wonder Bread strategy of supplementation to junk food in its purest form. (Wonder Soda?) The big money has always been in processing foods, not selling them whole, and the industry's investment in the reductionist approach to food is probably safe. The fact is, there is something in us that loves a refined carbohydrate, and that something is the human brain. The human brain craves carbohydrates reduced to their energy essence, which is to say pure glucose. Once industry figured out how to transform the seeds of grasses into the chemical equivalent of sugar, there was probably no turning back.

And then of course there is sugar itself, the ultimate refined carbohydrate, which began flooding the marketplace and the human metabolism around the same time as refined flour. In 1874, England lifted its tariffs on imported sugar, the price dropped by half, and by the end of the nineteenth century fully a sixth of the calories in the English diet were coming from sugar, with much of the rest coming from refined flour.

With the general availability of cheap pure sugar, the human metabolism now had to contend not only with a constant flood of glucose, but also with more fructose than it had ever before encountered, because sugar

— sucrose — is half fructose.* (Per capita fructose consumption has increased 25 percent in the past thirty years.) In the natural world, fructose is a rare and precious thing, typically encountered seasonally in ripe fruit, when it comes packaged in a whole food full of fiber (which slows its absorption) and valuable micronutrients. It's no wonder we've been hardwired by natural selection to prize sweet foods: Sugar as it is ordinarily found in nature — in fruits and some vegetables — gives us a slow-release form of energy accompanied by minerals and all sorts of crucial micronutrients we can get nowhere else. (Even in honey, the purest form of sugar found in nature, you find some valuable micronutrients.)

One of the most momentous changes in the American diet since 1909 (when the USDA first began keeping track) has been the increase in the percentage of calories coming from sugars, from 13 percent to 20

---

*Fructose is metabolized differently from glucose; the body doesn't respond to it by producing insulin to convey it into cells to be used as energy. Rather, it is metabolized in the liver, which turns it first into glucose and then, if there is no call for glucose, into triglycerides — fat.

percent. Add to that the percentage of calories coming from carbohydrates (roughly 40 percent, or ten servings, nine of which are refined) and Americans are consuming a diet that is at least half sugars in one form or another — calories providing virtually nothing but energy. The energy density of these refined carbohydrates contributes to obesity in two ways. First, we consume many more calories per unit of food; the fiber that's been removed from these foods is precisely what would have made us feel full and stop eating. Also, the flash flood of glucose causes insulin levels to spike and then, once the cells have taken all that glucose out of circulation, drop precipitously, making us think we need to eat again.

While the widespread acceleration of the Western diet has given us the instant gratification of sugar, in many people — especially those newly exposed to it — the speediness of this food overwhelms the ability of insulin to process it, leading to type 2 diabetes and all the other chronic diseases associated with metabolic syndrome. As one nutrition expert put it to me, "We're in the middle of a national experiment in the mainlining of glucose." And don't forget the flood of fructose, which may represent an even greater evolutionary novelty, and therefore challenge to the human metabolism, than all that glucose.

It is probably no accident that rates of type 2 diabetes are lower among ethnic Europeans, who have had longer than other groups to accustom their metabolisms to fast-release refined carbohydrates: Their food environment changed first.[*] To encounter such a diet for the first time, as when people accustomed to a more traditional diet come to America or when fast food comes to them, delivers a shock to the system. This shock is what public health experts mean by the nutrition transition, and it can be deadly.

[*]In the past, changes in the food environment have led to measurable changes in human biology over time. A recent study found that populations eating a high-starch diet have more copies of a gene coding for amylase, the enzyme needed to break down starch. The authors of the study suggest that natural selection has favored the gene in those populations that began eating cereal grains after the birth of agriculture. George H. Perry, et al., "Diet and the Evolution of Human Amylase Gene Copy Number Variation," *Nature Genetics* published online September 9, 2007; doi:10.1038/ng2123.

So here, then, is the first momentous change in the Western diet that may help to explain why it makes some people so sick: Supplanting tested relationships to the whole foods with which we coevolved over many thousands of years, it asks our bodies now to relate to, and deal with, a very small handful of efficiently delivered nutrients that have been torn from their food context. Our ancient evolutionary relationship with the seeds of grasses and fruit of plants has given way, abruptly, to a rocky marriage with glucose and fructose.

2) From Complexity to Simplicity

At every level, from the soil to the plate, the industrialization of the food chain has involved a process of chemical and biological simplification. It starts with industrial fertilizers, which grossly simplify the biochemistry of the soil. In the wake of Liebig's identification of the big three macronutrients that plants need to grow — nitrogen, phosphorus, and potassium (NPK) — and Fritz Haber's invention of a method for synthesizing nitrogen fertilizer from fossil fuels, agricultural soils began receiving large doses of the big three but little else. Just like Liebig, whose focus on the macronutrients in the human diet failed to take account of the important role played by micronutrients such as vitamins, Haber completely overlooked the importance of biological activity in the soil: the contribution to plant health of the complex underground ecosystem of soil microbes, earthworms, and mycorrhizal fungi. Harsh chemical fertilizers (and pesticides) depress or destroy this biological activity, forcing crops to subsist largely on a simple ration of NPK. Plants can live on this fast-food diet of chemicals, but it leaves them more vulnerable to pests and diseases and appears to diminish their nutritional quality.

It stands to reason that a chemically simplified soil would produce chemically simplified plants. Since the widespread adoption of chemical fertilizers in the 1950s, the nutritional quality of produce in America has declined substantially, according to figures gathered by the USDA, which has tracked the nutrient content of various crops since then. Some researchers blame this decline on the condition of the soil; others cite the tendency of modern plant breeding, which has consistently selected for industrial characteristics such as yield rather than nutritional quality. (The next section will take up the trade-off between quality and quantity in industrial food.)

The trend toward simplification of our food continues up the chain. As we've seen, processing whole foods — refining, chemically preserving, and canning them — depletes them of many nutrients, a few of which are then added back: B vitamins in refined flour, vitamins and minerals in breakfast cereal and bread. Fortifying processed foods with missing nutrients is surely better than leaving them out, but food science can add back only the small handful of nutrients that food science recognizes as important today. What is it overlooking? As the whole-grain food synergy study suggests, science doesn't know nearly enough to compensate for everything that processing does to whole foods. We know how to break down a kernel of corn or grain of wheat into its chemical parts, but we have no idea how to put it back together again. Destroying complexity is a lot easier than creating it.

Simplification of the food chain occurs at the level of species diversity too. The astounding variety of foods on offer in today's supermarket obscures the fact that the actual number of species in the modern diet is shrinking. Thousands of plant and animal varieties have fallen out of commerce in the last century as industrial agriculture has focused its attentions on a small handful of high-yielding (and usually patented) varieties, with qualities that suited them to things like mechanical harvesting and processing. Half of all the broccoli grown commercially in America today is a single variety — Marathon — notable for its high yield. The overwhelming majority of the chickens raised for meat in America are the same hybrid, the Cornish cross; more than 99 percent of the turkeys are Broad-Breasted Whites.

With the rise of industrial agriculture, vast monocultures of a tiny group of plants, most of them cereal grains, have replaced the diversified farms that used to feed us. A century ago, the typical Iowa farm raised more than a dozen different plant and animal species: cattle, chickens, corn, hogs, apples, hay, oats, potatoes, cherries, wheat, plums, grapes, and pears. Now it raises only two: corn and soybeans. This simplification of the agricultural landscape leads directly to the simplification of the diet, which is now to a remarkable extent dominated by — big surprise — corn and soybeans. You may not think you eat a lot of corn and soybeans, but you do: 75 percent of the vegetable oils in your diet come from soy (representing 20 percent of your daily calories) and more than half of the sweeteners you consume come from corn (representing around 10 percent of daily calories).

Why corn and soy? Because these two plants are among nature's most efficient transformers of sunlight and chemical fertilizer into carbohydrate energy (in the case of corn) and fat and protein (in the case of soy) — if you want to extract the maximum amount of macronutrients from the American farm belt, corn and soy are the crops to plant. (It helps that the government pays farmers to grow corn and soy, subsidizing every bushel they produce.) Most of the corn and soy crop winds up in the feed of our food animals (simplifying *their* diets in unhealthy ways, as we'll see), but much of the rest goes into processed foods. The business model of the food industry is organized around "adding value" to cheap raw materials; its genius has been to figure out how to break these two big seeds down into their chemical building blocks and then reassemble them in myriad packaged food products. With the result that today corn contributes 554 calories a day to America's per capita food supply and soy another 257. Add wheat (768 calories) and rice (91) and you can see there isn't a whole lot of room left in the American stomach for any other foods.

Today these four crops account for two thirds of the calories we eat. When you consider that humankind has historically consumed some eighty thousand edible species, and that three thousand of these have been in widespread use, this represents a radical simplification of the human diet. Why should this concern us? Because humans are omnivores, requiring somewhere between fifty and a hundred different chemical compounds and elements in order to be healthy. It's hard to believe we're getting everything we need from a diet consisting largely of processed corn, soybeans, rice, and wheat.

3) From Quality to Quantity

While industrial agriculture has made tremendous strides in coaxing macronutrients — calories — from the land, it is becoming increasingly clear that these gains in food quantity have come at a cost to its quality. This probably shouldn't surprise us: Our food system has long devoted its energies to increasing yields and selling food as cheaply as possible. It would be too much to hope those goals could be achieved without sacrificing at least some of the nutritional quality of our food.

As mentioned earlier, USDA figures show a decline in the nutrient content of the forty-three crops it has tracked since the 1950s. In one recent analysis, vitamin C declined by 20 percent, iron by 15 percent, riboflavin by 38 percent, calcium by 16 percent. Government figures from England tell a similar story: declines since the fifties of 10 percent or more in levels of iron, zinc, calcium, and selenium across a range of food crops. To put this in more concrete terms, you now have to eat three apples to get the same amount of iron as you would have gotten from a single 1940 apple, and you'd have to eat several more slices of bread to get your recommended daily allowance of zinc than you would have a century ago.

These examples come from a 2007 report entitled "Still No Free Lunch" written by Brian Halweil, a researcher for Worldwatch, and published by the Organic Center, a research institute established by the organic food industry. "American agriculture's single-minded focus on increasing yields created a blind spot," Halweil writes, "where incremental erosion in the nutritional quality of our food . . . has largely escaped the notice of scientists, government, and consumers." The result is the nutritional equivalent of inflation, such that we have to eat more to get the same amount of various essential nutrients. The fact that at least 30 percent of Americans have a diet deficient in vitamin C, vitamin E, vitamin A, and magnesium surely owes more to eating processed foods full of empty calories than it does to lower levels of nutrients in the whole foods we aren't eating. Still, it doesn't help that the raw materials used in the manufacture of processed foods have declined in nutritional quality or that when we *are* eating whole foods, we're getting substantially less nutrition per calorie than we used to.[*]

Nutritional inflation seems to have two principal causes: changes in the way we grow food and changes in the kinds of foods we grow. Halweil cites a considerable body of research demonstrating that plants grown with industrial fertilizers are often nutritionally inferior to the same varieties grown in

[*]The news of declining nutrient levels in American produce prompted *The Packer,* a trade publication for the produce industry, to suggest that this might actually be good for business, because people would now need to eat more produce to get the same nutritional benefit.

organic soils. Why this should be so is uncertain, but there are a couple of hypotheses. Crops grown with chemical fertilizers grow more quickly, giving them less time and opportunity to accumulate nutrients other than the big three (nutrients in which industrial soils are apt to be deficient anyway). Also, easy access to the major nutrients means that industrial crops develop smaller and shallower root systems than organically grown plants; deeply rooted plants have access to more soil minerals. Biological activity in the soil almost certainly plays a role as well; the slow decomposition of organic matter releases a wide range of plant nutrients, possibly including compounds science hasn't yet identified as important. Also, a biologically active soil will have more mycorrhizae, the soil fungi that live in symbiosis with plant roots, supplying the plants with minerals in exchange for a ration of sugar.

In addition to these higher levels of minerals, organically grown crops have also been found to contain more phytochemicals — the various secondary compounds (including carotenoids and polyphenols) that plants produce in order to defend themselves from pests and diseases, many of which turn out to have important antioxidant, antiinflammatory, and other beneficial effects in humans. Because plants living on organic farms aren't sprayed with synthetic pesticides, they're forced to defend themselves, with the result that they tend to produce between 10 percent and 50 percent more of these valuable secondary compounds than conventionally grown plants.

Some combination of these environmental factors probably accounts for at least part of the decline in the nutritional quality of conventional crops, but genetics likely plays just as important a role. Very simply, we have been breeding crops for yield, not nutritional quality, and when you breed for one thing, you invariably sacrifice another. Halweil cites several studies demonstrating that when older crop varieties are grown side by side with modern cultivars, the older ones typically have lower yields but substantially higher nutrient levels. USDA researchers recently found that breeding to "improve" wheat varieties over the past 130 years (a period during which yields of grain per acre tripled) had reduced levels of iron by 28 percent and zinc and selenium by roughly a third. Similarly, milk from modern Holstein cows (in which breeders have managed to more than triple daily yield since 1950) has considerably less butterfat and other nutrients than that from older, less "improved" varieties like Jersey, Guernsey, and Brown Swiss.

Clearly the achievements of industrial agriculture have come at a cost: It can produce a great many more calories per acre, but each of those calories may supply less nutrition than it formerly did. And what has happened on the farm has happened in the food system as a whole as industry has pursued the same general strategy of promoting quantity at the expense of quality. You don't need to spend much time in an American supermarket to figure out that this is a food system organized around the objective of selling large quantities of calories as cheaply as possible.

Indeed, doing so has been official U.S. government policy since the mid-seventies, when a sharp spike in food prices brought protesting housewives into the street and prompted the Nixon administration to adopt an ambitious cheap food policy. Agricultural policies were rewritten to encourage farmers to plant crops like corn, soy, and wheat fencerow to fencerow, and it worked: Since 1980, American farmers have produced an average of 600 more calories per person per day, the price of food has fallen, portion sizes have ballooned, and, predictably, we're eating a whole lot more, at least 300 more calories a day than we consumed in 1985. What kind of calories? Nearly a quarter of these additional calories come from added sugars (and most of that in the form of high-fructose corn syrup); roughly another quarter from added fat (most of it in the form of soybean oil); 46 percent of them from grains (mostly refined); and the few calories left (8 percent) from fruits and vegetables.* The overwhelming majority of the calories Americans have added to their diets since 1985 — the 93 percent of them in the form of sugars, fats, and mostly refined grains — supply lots of energy but very little of anything else.

A diet based on quantity rather than quality has ushered a new creature onto the world stage: the human being who manages to be both overfed and undernourished, two characteristics seldom found in the same body in the long natural history of our species. In most traditional diets, when calories are adequate, nutrient intake will usually be adequate as well. Indeed, many traditional diets are nutrient rich and, at least com-

*These are USDA statistics from *FoodReview,* Vol. 25, Issue 3, a publication of the Economic Research Service at the USDA.

pared to ours, calorie poor. The Western diet has turned that relationship upside down. At a health clinic in Oakland, California, doctors report seeing overweight children suffering from old-time deficiency diseases such as rickets, long thought to have been consigned to history's dustheap in the developed world. But when children subsist on fast food rather than fresh fruits and vegetables and drink more soda than milk, the old deficiency diseases return — now even in the obese.

Bruce Ames, the renowned Berkeley biochemist, works with kids like this at Children's Hospital and Research Center in Oakland. He's convinced that our high-calorie, low-nutrient diet is responsible for many chronic diseases, including cancer. Ames has found that even subtle micronutrient deficiencies — far below the levels needed to produce acute deficiency diseases — can cause damage to DNA that may lead to cancer. Studying cultured human cells, he's found that "deficiency of vitamins C, E, B_{12}, B_6, niacin, folic acid, iron or zinc appears to mimic radiation by causing single- and double-strand DNA breaks, oxidative lesions, or both" — precursors to cancer. "This has serious implications, as half of the U.S. population may be deficient in at least one of these micronutrients." Most of the missing micronutrients are supplied by fruits and vegetables, of which only 20 percent of American children and 32 percent of adults eat the recommended five daily servings. The cellular mechanisms Ames has identified could explain why diets rich in vegetables and fruits seem to offer some protection against certain cancers.

Ames also believes, though he hasn't yet proven it, that micronutrient deficiencies may contribute to obesity. His hypothesis is that a body starved of critical nutrients will keep eating in the hope of obtaining them. The absence of these nutrients from the diet may "counteract the normal feeling of satiety after sufficient calories are eaten" and that such an unrelenting hunger "may be a biological strategy for obtaining missing nutrients." If Ames is right, then a food system organized around quantity rather than quality has a destructive feedback loop built into it, such that the more low-quality food one eats, the more one wants to eats, in a futile — but highly profitable — quest for the absent nutrient.

4) From Leaves to Seeds
It's no accident that the small handful of plants we've come to rely on are grains (soy

is a legume); these crops are exceptionally efficient at transforming sunlight, fertilizer, air, and water into macronutrients — carbohydrates, fats, and proteins. These macronutrients in turn can be profitably converted into meat, dairy, and processed foods of every description. Also, the fact that they come in the form of durable seeds which can be stored for long periods of time means they can function as commodities as well as foods, making these crops particularly well adapted to the needs of industrial capitalism.

The needs of the human eater are a very different matter, however. An oversupply of macronutrients, such as we now face, itself represents a serious threat to our health, as soaring rates of obesity and diabetes indicate. But, as the research of Bruce Ames and others suggests, the undersupply of micronutrients may constitute a threat just as grave. Put in the most basic terms, we're eating a lot more seeds and a lot fewer leaves (as do the animals we depend on), a tectonic dietary shift the full implications of which we are just now beginning to recognize. To borrow, again, the nutritionist's reductive vocabulary: Leaves provide a host of critical nutrients a body can't get from a diet of refined seeds. There are the antioxidants and phytochemicals; there is the fiber; and then there are the essential omega-3 fatty acids found in leaves, which some researchers believe will turn out to be the most crucial missing nutrient of all.

Most people associate omega-3 fatty acids with fish, but fish get them originally from green plants (specifically algae), which is where they all originate.* Plant leaves produce these essential fatty acids (we say they're essential because our bodies can't produce them on their own) as part of photosynthesis; they occupy the cell membranes of chloroplasts, helping them collect light. Seeds contain more of another kind of essential fatty acid, omega-6, which serves as a store of energy for the developing seedling. These two types of polyunsaturated fats perform very different functions in the plant as well as the plant eater. In describing their respective roles, I'm going to simplify the chemistry somewhat. For a more complete (and fascinating) account of

*Alpha-linolenic acid is the omega-3 fatty acid found in all green plants; it is the most common fat in nature. Fish contain even more valuable "long-chain" forms of omega-3, like EPA and DHA, which they get from the algae at the base of their food chain.

the biochemistry of these fats and the story of their discovery read Susan Allport's *The Queen of Fats.*[*]

Omega-3s appear to play an important role in neurological development and processing (the highest concentrations of omega-3s in humans are found in the tissues of the brain and the eyes), visual acuity (befitting their role in photosynthesis), the permeability of cell walls, the metabolism of glucose, and the calming of inflammation. Omega-6s are involved in fat storage (which is what they do for the plant), the rigidity of cell walls, clotting, and the inflammation response. It helps to think of omega-3s as fleet and flexible, omega-6s as sturdy and slow. Because the two fatty acids compete with each other for space in cell membranes and for the attention of various enzymes, the ratio between omega-3s and omega-6s, in the diet and in turn in our tissues, may matter more than the absolute quantity of either fat. So, too much omega-6 may be just as much a problem as too little omega-3.

[*]*The Queen of Fats: Why Omega-3s Were Removed from the Western Diet and What We Can Do to Replace Them* (Berkeley: University of California Press, 2006).

And that might well be a problem for people eating a Western diet. As the basis of our diet has shifted from leaves to seeds, the ratio of omega-6s to omega-3s in our bodies has changed too. The same is true for most of our food animals, which industrial agriculture has taken off their accustomed diet of green plants and put on a richer diet of seeds. The result has been a marked decline in the amount of omega-3s in modern meat, dairy products, and eggs, and an increase in the amount of omega-6s. At the same time, modern food production practices have further diminished the omega-3s in our diet. Omega-3s, being less stable than omega-6s, spoil more readily, so the food industry, focused on store food, has been strongly disposed against omega-3s long before we even knew what they were. (Omega-3s weren't recognized as essential to the human diet until the 1980s — some time after nutritionism's blanket hostility to fat had already taken hold.) For years plant breeders have been unwittingly selecting for plants that produce fewer omega-3s, because such crops don't spoil as quickly. (Wild greens like purslane have substantially higher levels of omega-3s than most domesticated plants.) Also, when food makers partially hydrogenate oils to render them more stable, it is the omega-3s that are eliminated. An executive from Frito-Lay told Susan Allport in no uncertain terms that because of their tendency to oxidize, omega-3s "cannot be used in processed foods."

Most of the official nutritional advice we've been getting since the 1970s has, again unwittingly, helped to push omega-3s out of the diet and to elevate levels of omega-6. Besides demonizing fats in general, that advice has encouraged us to move from saturated fats of animal origin (some of which, like butter, actually contain respectable amounts of omega-3s) to seed oils, most of which are much higher in omega-6s (corn oil especially), and even more so after partial hydrogenation. The move from butter (and especially butter from pastured cows) to margarine, besides introducing trans fats to the diet, markedly increased omega-6s at the cost of omega-3s.

Thus without even realizing what we were doing, we dramatically altered the ratio of these two essential fats in our diet and our bodies, with the result that the ratio of omega-6 to omega-3 in the typical American today stands at more than 10 to 1. Before the widespread introduction of seed oils at the turn of the last century, the ratio was closer to 3 to 1.

The precise role of these lipids in human health is still not completely understood, but some researchers are convinced that these historically low levels of omega-3 (or, conversely, historically high levels of omega-6) bear responsibility for many of the chronic diseases associated with the Western diet, including heart disease and diabetes. Population studies suggest that omega-3 levels in the diet are strongly correlated with rates of heart disease, stroke, and mortality from all causes.[*] For example, the Japanese, who consume large amounts of omega-3s (most of it in fish), have markedly low rates of cardiovascular disease in spite of their high rates of smoking and high blood pressure. Americans consume only a third as much omega-3s as the Japanese and have nearly four times the rate of death from heart disease. But there is more than epidemiology to link omega-3 levels and heart disease: Clinical studies have found that increasing the omega-3s in one's diet may reduce the chances of heart attack

[*]Joseph Hibbeln, et al., "Healthy Intakes of n-3 and n-6 Fatty Acids: Estimations Considering Worldwide Diversity," *American Journal of Clinical Nutrition,* 2006; 83 (suppl): 1483S–93S.

by a third.[*]

What biological mechanism could explain these findings? A couple of theories have emerged. Omega-3s are present in high concentrations in heart tissue where they seem to play a role in regulating heart rhythm and preventing fatal arrhythmias. Omega-3s also dampen the inflammation response, which omega-6s tend to excite. Inflammation is now believed to play an important role in cardiovascular disease as well as in a range of other disorders, including rheumatoid arthritis and Alzheimer's. Omega-6s supply the building blocks for a class of pro-inflammatory messenger chemicals involved in the body's rapid-response reaction to a range of problems. One of these compounds is thromboxane, which encourages blood platelets to aggregate into clots. In contrast, omega-3s slow the clotting response, which is probably why populations with particularly high levels of

[*]M. L. Daviglus, "Fish Consumption and the 30-Year Risk of Myocardial Infarction," *New England Journal of Medicine,* 1997; 336: 1046–53. K. W. Lee and G. Y. Lip, "The Role of Omega-3 Fatty Acids in the Secondary Prevention of Cardiovascular Disease," *QJM: An International Journal of Medicine,* 2003 July; 96(7):465–80.

omega-3s, such as the Inuit, are prone to bleeding. (If there is a danger to consuming too much omega-3, bleeding is probably it.)

The hypothesis that omega-3 might protect against heart disease was inspired by studies of Greenland Eskimos, in whom omega-3 consumption is high and heart disease rare. Eskimos eating their traditional marine-based diet also don't seem to get diabetes, and some researchers believe it is the omega-3s that protect them. Adding omega-3s to the diet of rats has been shown to protect them against insulin resistance. (The same effect has not been duplicated in humans, however.) The theory is that omega-3s increase the permeability of the cell's membranes and its rate of metabolism. (Hummingbirds have tons of omega-3s in their cell membranes; big mammals much less.) A cell with a rapid metabolism and permeable membrane should respond particularly well to insulin, absorbing more glucose from the blood to meet its higher energy requirements. That same mechanism suggests that diets high in omega-3s might protect against obesity as well.

So why is it, as Susan Allport writes, that "populations, when given the choice, will naturally drift toward foods with lesser amounts of omega-3s"? Because a faster metabolism increases the need for food and therefore the possibility of hunger, she suggests, which is a much less agreeable condition than being overweight. This might help explain why so many groups have adopted Western diets as soon as they get the chance.

It should be said that researchers working on omega-3s can sound a bit like Dr. Casaubon in *Middlemarch,* hard at work on his "Key to all Mythologies." Likewise, omega-3 researchers seem to be in possession of a Theory of Everything, including happiness. The same population studies that have correlated omega-3 deficiency to cardiovascular disease have also found strong correlations between falling levels of omega-3 in the diet and rising rates of depression, suicide, and even homicide. Some researchers implicate omega-3 deficiency in learning disabilities such as attention deficit disorder as well. That omega-3s play an important role in mental function has been recognized since the 1980s, when it was found that babies fed on infant formula supplemented with omega-3s scored significantly higher on tests of both mental development and visual acuity than babies receiving formula supplemented only with omega-6.

Could it be that the problem with the

Western diet is a gross deficiency in this essential nutrient? A growing number of researchers have concluded that it is, and they voice frustration that official nutritional advice has been slow to recognize the problem. To do so, of course, would mean conceding the error of past nutritional advice demonizing fats in general and promoting the switch to seed oils high in omega-6. But it seems likely that sooner or later the government will establish minimum daily requirements for omega-3 (several other governments already have) and, perhaps in time, doctors will routinely test us for omega-3 levels the way they already do for cholesterol.

Though maybe they should be testing for omega-6 levels as well, because it's possible that is the greater problem. Omega-6s exist in a kind of zero-sum relationship with omega-3s, counteracting most of the positive effects of omega-3 throughout the body. Merely adding omega-3s to the diet — by taking supplements, say — may not do much good unless we also reduce the high levels of omega-6s that have entered the Western diet with the advent of processed foods, seed oils, and foods from animals raised on grain. Nine percent of the calories in the American diet today come from a single omega-6 fatty acid: linoleic acid, most of it from soybean oil. Some nutrition experts think that this is fine: Omega-6s, after all, are essential fatty acids too, and their rise to dietary prominence has pushed out saturated fats, usually thought to be a positive development. But others strongly disagree, contending that the unprecedented proportion of omega-6s in the Western diet is contributing to the full range of disorders involving inflammation. Joseph Hibbeln, the researcher at the National Institutes of Health who conducted population studies correlating omega-3 consumption with everything from stroke to suicide, says that the billions we spend on antiinflammatory drugs such as aspirin, ibuprofen, and acetaminophen is money spent to undo the effects of too much omega-6 in the diet. He writes, "The increases in world [omega-6] consumption over the past century may be considered a very large uncontrolled experiment that may have contributed to increased societal burdens of aggression, depression, and cardiovascular mortality."[*]

[*]Joseph Hibbeln, et al., "Healthy Intakes of n-3 and n-6 Fatty Acids: Estimations Considering Worldwide Diversity," *American Journal of Clinical Nutrition,* 2006; 83 (suppl): 1483S–93S.

■ ■ ■ ■

Of all the changes to our food system that go under the heading "The Western Diet," the shift from a food chain with green plants at its base to one based on seeds may be the most far reaching of all. Nutritional scientists focus on different nutrients — whether the problem with modern diets is too many refined carbohydrates, not enough good fats, too many bad fats, or a deficiency of any number of micronutrients or too many total calories. But at the root of all these biochemical changes is a single ecological change. For the shift from leaves to seeds affects much more than the levels of omega-3 and omega-6 in the body. It also helps account for the flood of refined carbohydrates in the modern diet *and* the drought of so many micronutrients *and* the surfeit of total calories. *From leaves to seeds:* It's almost, if not quite, a Theory of Everything.

5) From Food Culture to Food Science

The last important change wrought by the Western diet is not, strictly speaking, ecological, at least not in any narrow sense of the word. But the industrialization of our food that we call the Western diet is systematically and deliberately undermining tradi-

184

tional food cultures everywhere. This may be as destructive of our health as any nutritional deficiency.

Before the modern food era — and before the rise of nutritionism — people relied for guidance about what to eat on their national or ethnic or regional cultures. We think of culture as a set of beliefs and practices to help mediate our relationship to other people, but of course culture — at least before the rise of modern science — has also played a critical role in helping to mediate people's relationship to nature. Eating being one of the most important manifestations of that relationship, cultures have had a great deal to say about what and how and why and when and how much we should eat. Of course when it comes to food, culture is another word for mom, the figure who typically passes on the food ways of the group — food ways that endured, by the way, only because they tended to keep people healthy.

The sheer novelty and glamour of the Western diet, with its seventeen thousand new food products every year and the marketing power — thirty-two billion dollars a year — used to sell us those products, has overwhelmed the force of tradition and left us where we now find ourselves: relying on science and journalism and government and marketing to help us decide what to eat. Nutritionism, which arose to help us better deal with the problems of the Western diet, has largely been co-opted by it: used by the industry to sell more nutritionally "enhanced" processed food and to undermine further the authority of traditional food cultures that stand in the way of fast food. Industry greatly amplifies the claims of nutritional science through its advertising and, through its sponsorship of self-serving nutritional research, corrupts it.[*] The predictable result is the general cacophony of nutritional information ringing in our ears and the widespread confusion that has come to surround this most funda-

[*]Several studies have found that when industry funds nutrition research, the conclusions are more likely to produce findings favorable to that industry's products. One such previously cited study, published by the Public Library of Science, is "Relationships Between Funding Source and Conclusion Among Nutrition-Related Scientific Articles," by David S. Ludwig, et al. See also Marion Nestle's *Food Politics: How the Food Industry Influences Nutrition and Health.* Revised edition. (Berkeley: University of California Press, 2007).

mental of creaturely activities: finding something good to eat.

You would not have bought this book and read this far into it if your food culture was intact and healthy. And while it is true that most of us unthinkingly place the authority of science above culture in all matters having to do with our health, that prejudice should at least be examined. The question we need to ask is, Are we better off with these new authorities telling us how to eat than we were with the traditional authorities they supplanted? The answer by now should be clear.

It might be argued that at this point we should simply accept that fast food *is* our food culture and get on with it. Over time, people will get used to eating this way, and our health will improve as we gradually adjust to the new food environment. Also, as nutritional science improves, we should be able to ameliorate the worst effects of this diet. Already food scientists are figuring out ways to microencapsulate omega-3s and bake them into our vitamin-fortified bread. But I'm not sure we should put our faith in food science, which so far has not served us very well, or in evolution, either.

There are a couple of problems with trying simply to get used to the Western diet.

You could argue that, compared to the Aborigines, say, or Inuit, we *are* getting used to it — most of us don't get quite as fat or diabetic as they do. But our "adjustment" looks much less plausible when you consider that, as mentioned, fully a quarter of all Americans suffer from metabolic syndrome, two thirds of us are overweight or obese, and diet-related diseases are already killing the majority of us. The concept of a changing food environment is not just a metaphor; nor is the idea of adapting to it. In order for natural selection to help us adapt to the Western diet, we'd have to be prepared to let those whom it sickens die. Also, many of the chronic diseases caused by the Western diet come late in life, after the childbearing years, a period of our lives in which natural selection takes no interest. Thus genes predisposing people to these conditions get passed on rather than weeded out.

So we turn for salvation to the health care industry. Medicine is learning how to keep alive the people whom the Western diet is making sick. Doctors have gotten really good at keeping people with heart disease alive, and now they're hard at work on obesity and diabetes. Much more so than the human body, capitalism is marvelously adaptive, able to turn the problems it creates into new business opportunities: diet pills, heart bypass operations, insulin pumps, bariatric surgery. But though fast food may be good business for the health care industry, the cost to society — an estimated $250 billion a year in diet-related health care costs and rising rapidly — cannot be sustained indefinitely. An American born in 2000 has a 1 in 3 chance of developing diabetes in his lifetime; the risk is even greater for a Hispanic American or African American. A diagnosis of diabetes subtracts roughly twelve years from one's life and living with the condition incurs medical costs of $13,000 a year (compared with $2,500 for someone without diabetes).

This is a global pandemic in the making, but a most unusual one, because it involves no virus or bacteria, no microbe of any kind — just a way of eating. It remains to be seen whether we'll respond by changing our diet or our culture and economy. Although an estimated 80 percent of cases of type 2 diabetes could be prevented by a change of diet and exercise, it looks like the smart money is instead on the creation of a vast new diabetes industry. The mainstream media is full of advertisements for new gadgets and drugs for diabetics, and the health care industry is gearing up to meet the surging demand for heart bypass operations (80 percent of diabetics will suffer from heart disease), dialysis, and kidney transplantation. At the supermarket checkout you can thumb copies of a new lifestyle magazine, *Diabetic Living*. Diabetes is well on its way to becoming normalized in the West — recognized as a whole new demographic and so a major marketing opportunity. Apparently it is easier, or at least a lot more profitable, to change a disease of civilization into a lifestyle than it is to change the way that civilization eats.

■ ■ ■ ■

III
GETTING OVER
NUTRITIONISM

■ ■ ■ ■

One:
Escape from the Western Diet

The undertow of nutritionism is powerful, and more than once over the past few pages I've felt myself being dragged back under. You've no doubt noticed that much of the nutrition science I've presented here qualifies as reductionist science, focusing as it does on individual nutrients (such as certain fats or carbohydrates or antioxidants) rather than on whole foods or dietary patterns. Guilty. But using this sort of science to try to figure out what's wrong with the Western diet is probably unavoidable. However imperfect, it's the sharpest experimental and explanatory tool we have. It also satisfies our hunger for a simple, one-nutrient explanation. Yet it's one thing to entertain such explanations and quite another to mistake them for the whole truth or to let any one of them dictate the way you eat.

You've probably also noticed that many of the scientific theories put forward to account for exactly what in the Western diet is responsible for Western diseases conflict with one another. The lipid hypothesis cannot be reconciled with the carbohydrate hypothesis, and the theory that a deficiency of omega-3 fatty acids (call it the neolipid hypothesis) is chiefly to blame for chronic illness is at odds with the theory that refined carbohydrates are the key. And while everyone can agree that the flood of refined carbohydrates has pushed important micronutrients out of the modern diet, the scientists who blame our health problems on deficiencies of these micronutrients are not the same scientists who see a sugar-soaked diet leading to metabolic syndrome and from there to diabetes, heart disease, and cancer. It is only natural for scientists no less than the rest of us to gravitate toward a single, all-encompassing explanation. That is probably why you now find some of the most fervent critics of the lipid hypothesis embracing the carbohydrate hypothesis with the same absolutist zeal that they once condemned in the Fat Boys. In the course of my own research into these theories, I have been specifically warned by scientists allied with the carbohydrate camp not to "fall under the spell of the omega-3 cult." *Cult?* There is a lot more religion in science than you might expect.

So here we find ourselves once again, lost at sea amid the crosscurrents of conflicting science.

Or do we?

Because it turns out we don't need to declare our allegiance to any one of these schools of thought in order to figure out how best to eat. In the end, they are only theories, scientific explanations for an empirical phenomenon that is not itself in doubt: People eating a Western diet are prone to a complex of chronic diseases that seldom strike people eating more traditional diets. Scientists can argue all they want about the biological mechanisms behind this phenomenon, but whichever it is, the solution to the problem would appear to remain very much the same: *Stop eating a Western diet.*

In truth the chief value of any and all theories of nutrition, apart from satisfying our curiosity about how things work, is not to the eater so much as it is to the food industry and the medical community. The food industry needs theories so it can better redesign specific processed foods; a new theory means a new line of products, allowing the industry to go on tweaking the Western diet instead of making any more radical change to its business model. For the industry it's obviously preferable to have a scientific rationale for *further* processing foods — whether by lowering the fat or carbs or by boosting omega-3s or fortifying them with antioxidants and probiotics — than to entertain seriously the proposition that processed foods of any kind are a big part of the problem.

For the medical community too scientific theories about diet nourish business as usual. New theories beget new drugs to treat diabetes, high blood pressure, and cholesterol; new treatments and procedures to ameliorate chronic diseases; and new diets organized around each new theory's elevation of one class of nutrient and demotion of another. Much lip service is paid to the importance of prevention, but the health care industry, being an industry, stands to profit more handsomely from new drugs and procedures to treat chronic diseases than it does from a wholesale change in the way people eat. Cynical? Perhaps. You could argue that the medical community's willingness to treat the broad contours of the Western diet as a given is a reflection of its realism rather than its greed. "People don't want to go there," as Walter Willett responded to the critic who asked him why the Nurses' Health Study didn't study the benefits of more alternative diets. Still, medicalizing the whole problem of the Western diet instead of working to overturn it (whether at the level of the patient or politics) is exactly what you'd expect from a health care community that is sympathetic to nutritionism as a matter of temperament, philosophy, and economics. You would not expect such a medical community to be sensitive to the cultural or ecological dimensions of the food problem — and it isn't. We'll know this has changed when doctors kick the fast-food franchises out of the hospitals.

So what would a more ecological or cultural approach to the food problem counsel us? How might we plot our escape from nutritionism and, in turn, from the most harmful effects of the Western diet? To Denis Burkitt, the English doctor stationed in Africa during World War II who gave the Western diseases their name, the answer seemed straightforward, if daunting. "The only way we're going to reduce disease," he said, "is to go backwards to the diet and lifestyle of our ancestors." This sounds uncomfortably like the approach of the diabetic Aborigines who went back to the bush to heal themselves. But I don't think this is what Burkitt had in mind; even if it was, it is not a very attractive or practical strategy for most of us. No, the challenge we face today is figuring out how to escape the worst elements of the Western diet and lifestyle *without* going back to the bush.

In theory, nothing could be simpler: To escape the Western diet and the ideology of nutritionism, we have only to stop eating and thinking that way. But this is harder to do in practice, given the treacherous food environment we now inhabit and the loss of cultural tools to guide us through it. Take the question of whole versus processed foods, presumably one of the simpler distinctions between modern industrial foods and older kinds. Gyorgy Scrinis, who coined the term "nutritionism," suggests that the most important fact about any food is not its nutrient content but its degree of processing. He writes that "whole foods and industrial foods are the only two food groups I'd consider including in any useful food 'pyramid.' " In other words, instead of worrying about nutrients, we should simply avoid any food that has been processed to such an extent that it is more the product of industry than of nature.

This sounds like a sensible rule of thumb until you realize that industrial processes have by now invaded many whole foods too. Is a steak from a feedlot steer that consumed a diet of corn, various industrial waste products, antibiotics, and hormones still a "whole food"? I'm not so sure. The steer has itself been raised on a Western diet, and that diet has rendered its meat substantially different — in the type and amount of fat in it as well as its vitamin content — from the beef our ancestors ate. The steer's industrial upbringing has also rendered its meat so cheap that we're likely to eat more of it more often than our ancestors ever would have. This suggests yet another sense in which this beef has become an industrial food: It is designed to be eaten industrially too — as fast food.

So plotting our way out of the Western diet is not going to be simple. Yet I am convinced that it can be done, and in the course of my research, I have collected and developed some straightforward (and distinctly unscientific) rules of thumb, or personal eating policies, that might at least point us in the right direction. They don't say much about specific foods — about what sort of oil to cook with or whether you should eat meat. They don't have much to say about nutrients or calories, either, though eating according to these rules will perforce change the balance of nutrients and amount of calories in your diet. I'm not interested in dictating anyone's menu, but rather in developing what I think of as eating algorithms — mental programs that, if you run them when you're shopping for food or deciding on a meal, will produce a great many different dinners, all of them "healthy" in the broadest sense of that word.

And our sense of that word stands in need of some broadening. When most of us think about food and health, we think in fairly narrow nutritionist terms — about our personal physical health and how the ingestion of this particular nutrient or rejection of that affects it. But I no longer think it's possible to separate our bodily health from the health of the environment from which we eat or the environment in which we eat or, for that matter, from the health of our general outlook about food (and health). If my explorations of the food chain have taught me anything, it's that it *is* a food chain, and all the links in it are in fact linked: the health of the soil to the health of the plants and animals we eat to the health of the food culture in which we eat them to the health of the eater, in body as well as mind. So you will find rules here concerning not only what to eat but also how to eat it as well as how that food is produced. Food consists not just in piles of chemicals; it also comprises a set of social and ecological relationships, reaching back to the land and outward to other people. Some of these rules may strike you as having nothing whatever to do with health; in fact they do.

Many of the policies will also strike you as involving more work — and in fact they do. If there is one important sense in which we do need to heed Burkitt's call to "go backwards" or follow the Aborigines back into the bush, it is this one: In order to eat well we need to invest more time, effort, and resources in providing for our sustenance, to dust off a word, than most of us do today. A hallmark of the Western diet is food that is fast, cheap, and easy. Americans spend less than 10 percent of their income on food; they also spend less than a half hour a day preparing meals and little more than an hour enjoying them.[*] For most people for

*David M. Cutler, et al., "Why Have Americans Become More Obese?," *Journal of Economic Perspectives,* Vol. 17, No. 3 (Summer, 2003), pp. 93–118. In 1995 Americans spent twenty-seven minutes preparing meals and four minutes cleaning up after them; in 1965 the figure was forty-four minutes of preparation and twenty-one

most of history, gathering and preparing food has been an occupation at the very heart of daily life. Traditionally people have allocated a far greater proportion of their income to food — as they still do in several of the countries where people eat better than we do and as a consequence are healthier than we are.* Here, then, is one way in which we would do well to go a little native: backward, or perhaps it is forward, to a time and place where the gathering and preparing and enjoying of food were closer to the center of a well-lived life.

This book started out with seven words and three rules — *"Eat food. Not too much. Mostly plants"* — that I now need to unpack, providing some elaboration and refinement in the form of more specific guidelines, injunctions, subclauses, and the like. Each of these three main rules can serve as

---

minutes of cleanup. Total time spent eating has dropped from sixty-nine minutes to sixty-five, all of which suggests a trend toward prepackaged meals.

*Compared to the 9.9 percent of their income Americans spend on food, the Italians spend 14.9 percent, the French 14.9 percent, and the Spanish 17.1 percent.

category headings for a set of personal policies to guide us in our eating choices without too much trouble or thought. The idea behind having a simple policy like "avoid foods that make health claims" is to make the process simpler and more pleasurable than trying to eat by the numbers and nutrients, as nutritionism encourages us to do.

So under "Eat Food," I propose some practical ways to separate, and defend, real food from the cascade of foodlike products that now surround and confound us, especially in the supermarket. Many of the tips under this rubric concern shopping and take the form of filters that should help keep out the sort of products you want to avoid. Under "Mostly Plants," I'll dwell more specifically, and affirmatively, on the best types of foods (not nutrients) to eat. Lest you worry, there is, as the adverb suggests, more to this list than fruits and vegetables. Last, under "Not Too Much," the focus shifts from the foods themselves to the question of how to eat them — the manners, mores, and habits that go into creating a healthy, and pleasing, culture of eating.

Two:
Eat Food: Food Defined

The first time I heard the advice to "just eat food" it was in a speech by Joan Gussow, and it completely baffled me. Of course you should eat food — what else *is* there to eat? But Gussow, who grows much of her own food on a flood-prone finger of land jutting into the Hudson River, refuses to dignify most of the products for sale in the supermarket with that title. "In the thirty-four years I've been in the field of nutrition," she said in the same speech, "I have watched real food disappear from large areas of the supermarket and from much of the rest of the eating world." Taking food's place on the shelves has been an unending stream of foodlike substitutes, some seventeen thousand new ones every year — "products constructed largely around commerce and hope, supported by frighteningly little actual knowledge." Ordinary food is still out there, however, still being grown and even occasionally sold in the supermarket, and this ordinary food is what we should eat.

But given our current state of confusion and given the thousands of products calling themselves food, this is more easily said than done. So consider these related rules of thumb. Each proposes a different sort of map to the contemporary food landscape, but all should take you to more or less the same place.

Don't eat anything your great grandmother wouldn't recognize as food. Why your great grandmother? Because at this point your mother and possibly even your grandmother is as confused as the rest of us; to be safe we need to go back at least a couple generations, to a time before the advent of most modern foods. So depending on your age (and your grandmother), you may need to go back to your great- or even great-great grandmother. Some nutritionists recommend going back even further. John Yudkin, a British nutritionist whose early alarms about the dangers of refined carbohydrates were overlooked in the 1960s and 1970s, once advised, "Just don't eat anything your Neolithic ancestors wouldn't have recognized and you'll be ok."

What would shopping this way mean in the supermarket? Well, imagine your great grandmother at your side as you roll down the aisles. You're standing together in front of the dairy case. She picks up a package of Go-Gurt Portable Yogurt tubes — and has no idea what this could possibly be. Is it a food or a toothpaste? And how, exactly, do you introduce it into your body? You could tell her it's just yogurt in a squirtable form, yet if she read the ingredients label she would have every reason to doubt that that was in fact the case. Sure, there's some yogurt in there, but there are also a dozen other things that aren't remotely yogurtlike, ingredients she would probably fail to recognize as foods of any kind, including high-fructose corn syrup, modified corn starch, kosher gelatin, carrageenan, tricalcium phosphate, natural and artificial flavors, vitamins, and so forth. (And there's a whole other list of ingredients for the "berry bubblegum bash" flavoring, containing everything but berries or bubblegum.) How did yogurt, which in your great grandmother's day consisted simply of milk inoculated with a bacterial culture, ever get to be so complicated? Is a product like Go-Gurt Portable Yogurt still a whole food? A food of any kind? Or is it just a food product?

There are in fact hundreds of foodish products in the supermarket that your ancestors simply wouldn't recognize as food: breakfast cereal bars transected by bright white veins representing, but in reality having nothing to do with, milk; "protein waters" and "nondairy creamer"; cheeselike foodstuffs equally innocent of any bovine contribution; cakelike cylinders (with creamlike fillings) called Twinkies that never grow stale. *Don't eat anything incapable of rotting* is another personal policy you might consider adopting.

There are many reasons to avoid eating such complicated food products beyond the various chemical additives and corn and soy derivatives they contain. One of the problems with the products of food science is that, as Joan Gussow has pointed out, they lie to your body; their artificial colors and flavors and synthetic sweeteners and novel fats confound the senses we rely on to assess new foods and prepare our bodies to deal with them. Foods that lie leave us with little choice but to eat by the numbers, consulting labels rather than our senses.

It's true that foods have long been processed in order to preserve them, as when we pickle or ferment or smoke, but industrial processing aims to do much more than extend shelf life. Today foods are processed in ways specifically designed to sell us more food by pushing our evolutionary buttons — our inborn preferences for sweetness and fat and salt. These qualities are difficult to find in nature but cheap and easy for the food scientist to deploy, with the result that processing induces us to consume much more of these ecological rarities than is good for us. "Tastes great, less filling!" could be the motto for most processed foods, which are far more energy dense than most whole foods: They contain much less water, fiber, and micronutrients, and generally much more sugar and fat, making them at the same time, to coin a marketing slogan, "More fattening, less nutritious!"

The great grandma rule will help keep many of these products out of your cart. But not all of them. Because thanks to the FDA's willingness, post–1973, to let food makers freely alter the identity of "traditional foods that everyone knows" without having to call them imitations, your great grandmother could easily be fooled into thinking that that loaf of bread or wedge of cheese is in fact a loaf of bread or a wedge of cheese. This is why we need a slightly more detailed personal policy to capture these imitation foods; to wit:

Avoid food products containing ingredients that are a) unfamiliar, b) unpronounceable, c) more than five in number, or that include d) high-fructose corn syrup. None of these characteristics, not even the last one, is necessarily harmful in and of itself, but all of them are reliable markers for foods that have been highly processed to the point where they may no longer be what they purport to be. They have crossed over from foods to food products.

Consider a loaf of bread, one of the "traditional foods that everyone knows" specifically singled out for protection in the 1938 imitation rule. As your grandmother could tell you, bread is traditionally made using a remarkably small number of familiar ingredients: flour, yeast, water, and a pinch of salt will do it. But industrial bread — even industrial whole-grain bread — has become a far more complicated product of modern food science (not to mention commerce and hope). Here's the complete ingredients list for Sara Lee's Soft & Smooth Whole Grain White Bread. (Wait a minute — isn't "Whole Grain White Bread" a contradiction in terms? Evidently not any more.)

Enriched bleached flour [wheat flour, malted barley flour, niacin, iron, thiamin mononitrate (vitamin B_1), riboflavin (vitamin B_2), folic acid], water, whole grains [whole wheat flour, brown rice flour (rice flour, rice bran)], high fructose corn *syrup [hello!], whey, wheat gluten, yeast, cellulose. Contains 2% or less of each of the following: honey, calcium sulfate, vegetable oil (soybean and/or cottonseed oils), salt, butter (cream, salt), dough conditioners (may contain one or more of the following: mono- and diglycerides, ethoxylated mono- and diglycerides, ascorbic acid, enzymes, azodicarbonamide), guar gum, calcium propionate (preservative), distilled vinegar, yeast nutrients (monocalcium phosphate, calcium sulfate, ammonium sulfate), corn starch, natural flavor, beta-carotene (color), vitamin D$_3$, soy lecithin, soy flour.*

There are many things you could say about this intricate loaf of "bread," but note first that even if it managed to slip by your great grandmother (because it *is* a loaf of bread, or at least is called one and strongly resembles one), the product fails every test proposed under rule number two: It's got unfamiliar ingredients (monoglycerides I've heard of before, but ethoxylated monoglycerides?); unpronounceable ingredients (try "azodicarbonamide"); it exceeds the maximum of five ingredients (by roughly thirty-six); and it contains high-fructose corn syrup. Sorry, Sara Lee, but your Soft

& Smooth Whole Grain White Bread is not food and if not for the indulgence of the FDA could not even be labeled "bread."

Sara Lee's Soft & Smooth Whole Grain White Bread could serve as a monument to the age of nutritionism. It embodies the latest nutritional wisdom from science and government (which in its most recent food pyramid recommends that at least half our consumption of grain come from whole grains) but leavens that wisdom with the commercial recognition that American eaters (and American children in particular) have come to prefer their wheat highly refined — which is to say, cottony soft, snowy white, and exceptionally sweet on the tongue. In its marketing materials, Sara Lee treats this clash of interests as some sort of Gordian knot — it speaks in terms of an ambitious quest to build a "no compromise" loaf — which only the most sophisticated food science could possibly cut.

And so it has, with the invention of whole-grain white bread. Because the small percentage of whole grains in the bread would render it that much less sweet than, say, all-white Wonder Bread — which scarcely waits to be chewed before transforming itself into glucose — the food scientists have added high-fructose corn syrup and honey to make up the difference; to overcome the problematic heft and toothsomeness of a real whole grain bread, they've deployed "dough conditioners," including guar gum and the aforementioned azodicarbonamide, to simulate the texture of supermarket white bread. By incorporating certain varieties of albino wheat, they've managed to maintain that deathly but apparently appealing Wonder Bread pallor.

Who would have thought Wonder Bread would ever become an ideal of aesthetic and gustatory perfection to which bakers would actually aspire — Sara Lee's Mona Lisa?

Very often food science's efforts to make traditional foods more nutritious make them much more complicated, but not necessarily any better for you. To make dairy products low fat, it's not enough to remove the fat. You then have to go to great lengths to preserve the body or creamy texture by working in all kinds of food additives. In the case of low-fat or skim milk, that usually means adding powdered milk. But powdered milk contains oxidized cholesterol, which scientists believe is much worse for your arteries than ordinary cholesterol, so food makers sometimes compensate by adding antioxidants, further complicating what had been a simple one-ingredient whole food. Also, removing the fat makes it that much harder for your body to absorb the fat-soluble vitamins that are one of the reasons to drink milk in the first place.

All this heroic and occasionally counter-productive food science has been under-taken in the name of our health — so that Sara Lee can add to its plastic wrapper the magic words "good source of whole grain" or a food company can ballyhoo the even more magic words "low fat." Which brings us to a related food policy that may at first sound counterintuitive to a health-conscious eater:

Avoid food products that make health claims. For a food product to make health claims on its package it must first *have* a package, so right off the bat it's more likely to be a processed than a whole food. Generally speaking, it is only the big food companies that have the wherewithal to secure FDA-approved health claims for their products and then trumpet them to the world. Recently, however, some of the tonier fruits and nuts have begun boasting about their health-enhancing properties, and there will surely be more as each crop council scrounges together the money to commission its own scientific study. Because all plants contain antioxidants, all these studies are guaranteed to find *some*thing on which to base a health oriented marketing campaign.

But for the most part it is the products of food science that make the boldest health claims, and these are often founded on incomplete and often erroneous science — the dubious fruits of nutritionism. Don't forget that trans-fat-rich margarine, one of the first industrial foods to claim it was healthier than the traditional food it replaced, turned out to give people heart attacks. Since that debacle, the FDA, under tremendous pressure from industry, has made it only easier for food companies to make increasingly doubtful health claims, such as the one Frito-Lay now puts on some of its chips — that eating them is somehow good for your heart. If you bother to read the health claims closely (as food marketers make sure consumers seldom do), you will find that there is often considerably less to them than meets the eye.

Consider a recent "qualified" health claim approved by the FDA for (don't laugh) corn oil. ("Qualified" is a whole new category of health claim, introduced in 2002 at the behest of industry.) Corn oil, you may recall, is particularly high in the omega-6 fatty acids we're already consuming far too many of.

Very limited and preliminary scientific evidence suggests that eating about one tablespoon (16 grams) of corn oil daily may reduce the risk of heart disease due to the unsaturated fat content in corn oil.

The tablespoon is a particularly rich touch, conjuring images of moms administering medicine, or perhaps cod-liver oil, to their children. But what the FDA gives with one hand, it takes away with the other. Here's the small-print "qualification" of this already notably diffident health claim:

[The] FDA concludes that there is little scientific evidence supporting this claim.

And then to make matters still more perplexing:

To achieve this possible benefit, corn oil is to replace a similar amount of saturated fat and not increase the total number of calories you eat in a day.

This little masterpiece of pseudoscientific bureaucratese was extracted from the FDA by the manufacturer of Mazola corn oil. It would appear that "qualified" is an official FDA euphemism for "all but meaningless." Though someone might have let the consumer in on this game: The FDA's own research indicates that consumers have no idea what to make of qualified health claims (how would they?), and its rules allow companies to promote the claims pretty much any way they want — they can use really big type for the claim, for example, and then print the disclaimers in teeny-tiny type. No doubt we can look forward to a qualified health claim for high-fructose corn syrup, a tablespoon of which probably does contribute to your health — as long as it replaces a comparable amount of, say, poison in your diet and doesn't increase the total number of calories you eat in a day.

When corn oil and chips and sugary breakfast cereals can all boast being good for your heart, health claims have become hopelessly corrupt. The American Heart Association currently bestows (for a fee) its heart-healthy seal of approval on Lucky Charms, Cocoa Puffs, and Trix cereals, Yoo-hoo lite chocolate drink, and Healthy Choice's Premium Caramel Swirl Ice Cream Sandwich — this at a time when scientists are coming to recognize that dietary sugar probably plays a more important role in heart disease than dietary fat. Meanwhile, the genuinely heart-healthy whole foods in the produce section, lacking the financial and political clout of the packaged goods a few aisles over, are mute. But don't take the silence of the yams as a sign that they have nothing valuable to say about health.

Bogus health claims and food science have made supermarkets particularly treacherous places to shop for real food, which suggests two further rules:

Shop the peripheries of the supermarket and stay out of the middle. Most supermarkets are laid out the same way: Processed food products dominate the center aisles of the store while the cases of ostensibly fresh food — dairy, produce, meat, and fish — line the walls. If you keep to the edges of the store you'll be that much more likely to wind up with real food in your shopping cart. The strategy is not foolproof, however, because things like high-fructose corn syrup have slipped into the dairy case under cover of Go-Gurt and such. So consider a more radical strategy:

Get out of the supermarket whenever possible. You won't find *any* high-fructose corn

217

syrup at the farmers' market. You also won't find any elaborately processed food products, any packages with long lists of unpronounceable ingredients or dubious health claims, nothing microwavable, and, perhaps best of all, no old food from far away. What you *will* find are fresh whole foods picked at the peak of their taste and nutritional quality — precisely the kind your great grandmother, or even your Neolithic ancestors, would easily have recognized as food.

Indeed, the surest way to escape the Western diet is simply to depart the realms it rules: the supermarket, the convenience store, and the fast-food outlet. It is hard to eat badly from the farmers' market, from a CSA box (community-supported agriculture, an increasingly popular scheme in which you subscribe to a farm and receive a weekly box of produce), or from your garden. The number of farmers' markets has more than doubled in the last ten years, to more than four thousand, making it one of the fastest-growing segments of the food marketplace. It is true that most farmers' markets operate only seasonally, and you won't find everything you need there. But buying as much as you can from the farmers' market, or directly from the farm when that's an option, is a simple act with a host of profound consequences for your health as well as for the health of the food chain you've now joined.

When you eat from the farmers' market, you automatically eat food that is in season, which is usually when it is most nutritious. Eating in season also tends to diversify your diet — because you can't buy strawberries or broccoli or potatoes twelve months of the year, you'll find yourself experimenting with other foods when they come into the market. The CSA box does an even better job of forcing you out of your dietary rut because you'll find things in your weekly allotment that you would never buy on your own. Whether it's a rutabaga or an unfamiliar winter squash, the CSA box's contents invariably send you to your cookbooks to figure out what in the world to do with them. Cooking is one of the most important health consequences of buying food from local farmers; for one thing, when you cook at home you seldom find yourself reaching for the ethoxylated diglycerides or high-fructose corn syrup. But more on cooking later.

To shop at a farmers' market or sign up with a CSA is to join a short food chain and that has several implications for your health. Local produce is typically picked ripe and is fresher than supermarket produce, and for those reasons it should be tastier and more nutritious. As for supermarket organic produce, it too is likely to have come from far away — from the industrial organic farms of California or, increasingly, China.[*] And while it's true that the organic label guarantees that no synthetic pesticides or fertilizers have been used to produce the food, many, if not most, of the small farms that supply farmers' markets are organic in everything but name. To survive in the farmers' market or CSA economy, a farm will need to be highly diversified, and a diversified farm usually has little need for pesticides; it's the big monocultures that can't survive without them.[†]

If you're concerned about chemicals in

---

[*]One recent study found that the average item of organic produce in the supermarket had actually traveled farther from the farm than the average item of conventional produce.

[†]Wendell Berry put the problem of monoculture with admirable brevity and clarity in his essay "The Pleasures of Eating": "But as scale increases, diversity declines; as diversity declines, so does health; as health declines, the dependence on drugs and chemicals necessarily increases."

your produce, you can simply ask the farmer at the market how he or she deals with pests and fertility and begin the sort of conversation between producers and consumers that, in the end, is the best guarantee of quality in your food. So many of the problems of the industrial food chain stem from its length and complexity. A wall of ignorance intervenes between consumers and producers, and that wall fosters a certain carelessness on both sides. Farmers can lose sight of the fact that they're growing food for actual eaters rather than for middlemen, and consumers can easily forget that growing good food takes care and hard work. In a long food chain, the story and identity of the food (Who grew it? Where and how was it grown?) disappear into the undifferentiated stream of commodities, so that the only information communicated between consumers and producers is a price. In a short food chain, eaters can make their needs and desires known to the farmer, and farmers can impress on eaters the distinctions between ordinary and exceptional food, and the many reasons why exceptional food is worth what it costs. Food reclaims its story, and some of its nobility, when the person who grew it hands it to you. So here's a subclause to the get-out-of-the-supermarket rule: *Shake the hand that feeds you.*

As soon as you do, accountability becomes once again a matter of relationships instead of regulation or labeling or legal liability. Food safety didn't become a national or global problem until the industrialization of the food chain attenuated the relationships between food producers and eaters. That was the story Upton Sinclair told about the Beef Trust in 1906, and it's the story unfolding in China today, where the rapid industrialization of the food system is leading to alarming breakdowns in food safety and integrity. Regulation is an imperfect substitute for the accountability, and trust, built into a market in which food producers meet the gaze of eaters and vice versa. Only when we participate in a short food chain are we reminded every week that we are indeed part of a food chain and dependent for our health on its peoples and soils and integrity — on *its* health.

"Eating is an agricultural act," Wendell Berry famously wrote, by which he meant that we are not just passive consumers of food but cocreators of the systems that feed us. Depending on how we spend them, our food dollars can either go to support a food industry devoted to quantity and convenience and "value" or they can nourish a food chain organized around *values* — values like quality and health. Yes, shopping this way takes more money and effort, but as soon you begin to treat that expenditure not just as shopping but also as a kind of vote — a vote for health in the largest sense — food no longer seems like the smartest place to economize.

THREE:
MOSTLY PLANTS: WHAT TO EAT

If you can manage to just eat food most of the time, *what*ever that food is, you'll probably be okay. One lesson that can be drawn from the striking diversity of traditional diets that people have lived on around the world is that it is possible to nourish ourselves from an astonishing range of different foods, so long as they are foods. There have been, and can be, healthy high-fat and healthy low-fat diets, so long as they're built around whole foods rather than highly processed food products. Yet there are some whole foods that are better than others, and some ways of producing them and then combining them in meals that are worth attending to. So this section proposes a handful of personal policies regarding what to eat, above and beyond "food."

Eat mostly plants, especially leaves. Scientists may disagree about what's so good about eating plants — Is it the antioxidants in them? The fiber? The omega-3 fatty acids? — but they do agree that plants are probably really good for you, and certainly can't hurt. In all my interviews with nutrition experts, the benefits of a plant-based diet provided the only point of universal consensus. Even nutrition scientists who have been chastened by decades of conflict and confusion about dietary advice would answer my question "So what are you still sure of?" with some variation on the recommendation to "eat more plants." (Though Marion Nestle was slightly more circumspect: "Certainly eating plants isn't harmful.")

That plants are good for humans to eat probably doesn't need much elaboration, but the story of vitamin C, an antioxidant we depend primarily on plants to supply us, points to the evolutionary reasons why this might have become the case. Way back in evolution, our ancestors possessed the biological ability to make vitamin C, an essential nutrient, from scratch. Like other antioxidants, vitamin C, or ascorbic acid, contributes to our health in at least two important ways. Several of the body's routine processes, including cell metabolism and the defense mechanism of inflammation, produce "oxygen radicals" — atoms of oxygen with an extra unpaired electron that make them particularly eager to react with other molecules in ways that can create all kinds of trouble. Free radicals have been implicated in a great many health problems, including cancer and the various problems associated with aging. (Free-radical production rises as you get older.) Antioxidants like vitamin C harmlessly absorb and stabilize these radicals before they can do their mischief.

But antioxidants do something else for us as well: They stimulate the liver to produce the enzymes necessary to break down the antioxidant itself, enzymes that, once produced, go on to break down other compounds as well, including whatever toxins happen to resemble the antioxidant. In this way antioxidants help detoxify dangerous chemicals, including carcinogens, and the more kinds of antioxidants in the diet, the more kinds of toxins the body can disarm. This is one reason why it's important to eat as many different kinds of plants as possible: They all have different antioxidants and so help the body eliminate different kinds of toxins. (It stands to reason that the more toxins there are in the environment, the more plants you should be eating.)

Animals can synthesize some of their own antioxidants, including, once upon a time, vitamin C. But there was so much vitamin C in our ancestors' plant-rich diet that over time we lost our ability to make the compound ourselves, perhaps because natural selection tends to dispense with anything superfluous that is metabolically expensive to produce. (The reason plants are such a rich source of antioxidants is that they need them to cope with all the pure oxygen produced during photosynthesis.) This was a happy development for the plants, of course, because it made humans utterly dependent upon them for an essential nutrient — which is why humans have been doing so much for the vitamin C producers ever since, spreading their genes and expanding their habitat. We sometimes think of sweetness as the linchpin of the reciprocal relationship between plants and people, but antioxidants like vitamin C play an equally important, if less perceptible, part.

So our biological dependence on plants goes back and runs deep, which makes it not at all surprising that eating them should be so good for us. There are literally scores of studies demonstrating that a diet rich in vegetables and fruits reduces the risk of dying from all the Western diseases. In countries where people eat a pound or more of fruits and vegetables a day, the rate of cancer is half what it is in the United States. We also know that vegetarians are less susceptible to most of the Western diseases, and as a consequence live longer than the rest of us. (Though near vegetarians — so-called flexitarians — are just as healthy as vegetarians.) Exactly *why* this should be so is not quite as clear as the fact that it is. The antioxidants in plants almost certainly are protective, but so may be the omega-3s (also essential nutrients that we can't produce ourselves) and the fiber and still other plant components and synergies as yet unrecognized; as the whole-grain study suggests, plant foods are apt to be more than the sum of their nutrient parts.

But the advantages of a plant-based diet probably go beyond whatever is in the plants: Because plant foods — with the exception of seeds — are less energy dense than most of the other things you might eat, by eating a plant-based diet you will likely consume fewer calories (which is itself protective against many chronic diseases). The seed exception suggests why it's important to eat more leaves than seeds; though unrefined seeds, including whole grains and nuts, can be very nutritious, they're high in calories, befitting their biological role as energy-storage devices. It's only when we begin refining plant seeds or eating them to the exclusion of the rest of the plant that we get into trouble.

So what about eating meat? Unlike plants, which we can't live without, we don't *need* to eat meat — with the exception of B_{12}, every nutrient found in meat can be obtained somewhere else. (And the tiny amount of B_{12} we need is not too hard to come by; it's found in all animal foods and is produced by bacteria, so you obtain B_{12} from eating dirty or decaying or fermented produce.) But meat, which humans have been going to heroic lengths to obtain and have been relishing for a very long time, is nutritious food, supplying all the essential amino acids as well as many vitamins and minerals, and I haven't found a compelling health reason to exclude it from the diet. (That's not to say there aren't good ethical or environmental reasons to do so.[*])

*Industrial meat production is notoriously brutal

That said, eating meat in the tremendous quantities we do (each American now consumes an average of two hundred pounds of meat a year) is probably not a good idea, especially when that meat comes from a highly industrialized food chain. Several studies point to the conclusion that the more meat there is in your diet — red meat especially — the greater your risk of heart disease and cancer. Yet studies of flexitarians suggest that small amounts of meat — less than one serving a day — don't appear to increase one's risk. Thomas Jefferson probably had the right idea when he recommended using meat more as a flavor principle than as a main course, treating it as a

---

to the animals and extravagantly wasteful of resources such as water, grain, as well as antibiotics; the industry is also one of the biggest contributors to water and air pollution. A 2006 report issued by the United Nations stated that the world's livestock generate more greenhouse gases than the entire transportation industry. Henning Steinfeld, et al. *Livestock's Long Shadow: Environmental Issues and Options.* A report published by the Food and Agriculture Organization of the United Nations (Rome: FAO, 2006). Available online at http://www.virtualcentre.org/en/library/keypub/longshad/A0701E00.htm.

"condiment for the vegetables."

What exactly it is in meat we need to worry about (the saturated fat? the type of iron? the carcinogens produced in curing and cooking it?) is unclear; the problem could be simply that eating lots of it pushes plants out of the diet. But eating too much industrial meat exposes us to more saturated fat, omega-6 fatty acids, growth hormones, and carcinogens than we probably want in our diet. Meat has both the advantages and disadvantages of being at the top of the food chain: It accumulates and concentrates many of the nutrients in the environment but also many of the toxins.

Meat offers a good proof of the proposition that the healthfulness of a food cannot be divorced from the health of the food chain that produced it — that the health of soil, plant, animal, and eater are all connected, for better or worse. Which suggests a special rule for people eating animal foods:

You are what what you eat eats too. That is, the diet of the animals we eat has a bearing on the nutritional quality, and healthfulness, of the food itself, whether it is meat or milk or eggs. This should be self-evident, yet it is a truth routinely overlooked by the industrial food chain in its quest to produce vast quantities of cheap animal protein. That quest has changed the diet of most of our food animals from plants to seeds, because animals grow faster and produce more milk and eggs on a high-energy diet of grain. But some of our food animals, such as cows and sheep, are ruminants that evolved to eat grass; if they eat too many seeds they become sick, which is why grain-fed cattle have to be given antibiotics. Even animals that do well on grain, such as chickens and pigs, are much healthier when they have access to green plants, and so, it turns out, are their meat and eggs.

For most of our food animals, a diet of grass means much healthier fats (more omega-3s and conjugated linoleic acid, or CLA; fewer omega-6s and saturated fat) in their meat, milk, and eggs, as well as appreciably higher levels of vitamins and antioxidants. Sometimes you can actually see the difference, as when butter is yellow or egg yolks bright orange: What you're seeing is the beta-carotene from fresh green grass. It's worth looking for pastured animal foods in the market and paying the premium they typically command. For though from the outside an industrial egg looks exactly like a pastured egg selling for several times as much, they are for all intents and purposes

231

two completely different foods.[*] So the rule about eating more leaves and fewer seeds applies not only to us but also to the animals in our food chain.

If you have the space, buy a freezer. When you find a good source of pastured meat, you'll want to buy it in quantity. Buying meat in bulk — a quarter of a steer, say, or a whole hog — is one way to eat well on a budget. Dedicated freezers are surprisingly inexpensive to buy and to operate, because they don't get opened nearly as often as the one attached to your refrigerator. A freezer will also encourage you to put up food from the farmers' market, allowing you to buy produce in bulk when it is at the height of its season, which is when it will be most abundant and therefore cheapest. And freez-

[*]"Free range" doesn't necessarily mean the chicken has had access to grass; many egg and broiler producers offer their chickens little more than a dirt yard where nothing grows. Look for the word "pastured." And in the case of beef, keep in mind that all cattle are grass fed until they get to the feedlot; "grass finished" or "100% grass fed" is what you want. For more on the nutritional benefits of pastured food and where to find it, go to eatwild.com.

ing (unlike canning) does not significantly diminish the nutritional value of produce.

Eat like an omnivore. Whether or not you eat any animal foods, it's a good idea to try to add some new species, and not just new foods, to your diet. The dazzling diversity of food products on offer in the supermarket is deceptive because so many of them are made from the same small handful of plants, and most of those — like the corn and soy and wheat — are seeds. The greater the diversity of species you eat, the more likely you are to cover all your nutritional bases.

But that is an argument from nutritionism, and there is a better one, one that takes a broader view of health. Biodiversity in the diet means more biodiversity in the fields. To shrink the monocultures that now feed us would mean farmers won't need to spray as much pesticide or chemical fertilizer, which would mean healthier soils, healthier plants and animals, and in turn healthier people. Your health isn't bordered by your body, and what's good for the soil is probably good for you too. Which brings us to a related rule:

Eat well-grown food from healthy soils. It

would have been much simpler to say "eat organic" because it is true that food certified organic is usually well grown in relatively healthy soils — soils that have been nourished by organic matter rather than synthetic fertilizers. Yet there are exceptional farmers and ranchers in America who for one reason or another are not certified organic and the food they grow should not be overlooked. Organic is important, but it's not the last word on how to grow food well.

Also, the supermarket today is brimming with processed organic food products that are little better, at least from the standpoint of health, than their conventional counterparts. Organic Oreos are not a health food. When Coca-Cola begins selling organic Coke, as it surely will, the company will have struck a blow for the environment perhaps, but not for our health. Most consumers automatically assume that the word "organic" is synonymous with health, but it makes no difference to your insulin metabolism if the high-fructose corn syrup in your soda is organic.

Yet the superiority of real food grown in healthy soils seems clear. There is now a small but growing body of empirical research to support the hypothesis, first advanced by Sir Albert Howard and J. I. Rodale, that soils rich in organic matter produce more nutritious food. Recently a handful of well-controlled comparisons of crops grown organically and conventionally have found appreciably higher levels of anti-oxidants, flavonoids, vitamins, and other nutrients in several of the organic crops. Of course after a few days riding cross-country in a truck the nutritional quality of any kind of produce will deteriorate, so ideally you want to look for food that is both organic *and* local.

Eat wild foods when you can. Two of the most nutritious plants in the world are weeds — lamb's quarters and purslane — and some of the healthiest traditional diets, such as the Mediterranean, make frequent use of wild greens. The fields and forests are crowded with plants containing higher levels of various phytochemicals than their domesticated cousins. Why? Because these plants have to defend themselves against pests and disease without any help from us, and because historically we've tended to select and breed crop plants for sweetness; many of the defensive compounds plants produce are bitter. Wild greens also tend to have higher levels of omega-3 fatty acids than their domesticated cousins, which have been selected to hold up longer after picking.

Wild animals too are worth adding to your diet when you have the opportunity. Wild game generally has less saturated fat and more omega-3 fatty acids than domesticated animals, because most of the wild animals we eat themselves eat a diverse diet of plants rather than grain. (The nutritional profile of grass-fed beef closely resembles that of wild game.) Wild fish generally have higher levels of omega-3s than farmed fish, which are often fed grain. To judge by the experience of fish-eating cultures like the Japanese, adding a few servings of wild fish to the diet each week may lower our risk of heart disease, prolong our lives, and even make us happier.[*]

Yet I hesitate to recommend eating wild foods because so many of them are endan-

[*]Joseph Hibbeln, et al., "Healthy Intakes of n-3 and n-6 Fatty Acids: Estimations Considering Worldwide Diversity," *American Journal of Clinical Nutrition* (2006): 83 (suppl): 1483s–93s; Hibbeln, et al., "Dietary Polyunsaturated Fatty Acids and Depression: When Cholesterol Does Not Satisfy." *American Journal of Clinical Nutrition* (1995): 62:1–9.

gered; many wild fish stocks are on the verge of collapse because of overfishing. Up to now, all the recommendations I've offered here pose no conflict between what's best for your health and what's best for the environment. Indeed, most of them support farming and ranching practices that improve the health of the land and the water. But not this one, sorry to say. There are not enough wild animals left for us all to be eating more of them (except perhaps deer and feral pigs), and certainly not enough wild fish. Fortunately, however, a few of the most nutritious fish species, including salmon, mackerel, sardines, and anchovies, are well managed and in some cases even abundant. Don't overlook those oily little fish.

Be the kind of person who takes supplements. We know that people who take supplements are generally healthier than the rest of us, and we also know that, in controlled studies, most of the supplements they take don't appear to work. Probably the supplement takers are healthier for reasons having nothing to do with the pills: They're typically more health conscious, better educated, and more affluent. So to the extent you can, be the *kind* of person who would take supplements, and then save your money.

That said, many of the nutrition experts I consulted recommend taking a multivitamin, especially as you get older. In theory at least, your diet should provide all the micronutrients you need to be healthy, especially if you're eating real food and lots of plants. After all, we evolved to obtain whatever our bodies need from nature and wouldn't be here if we couldn't. But natural selection takes little interest in our health or survival after the childbearing years are past, and as we age our need for antioxidants increases while our bodies' ability to absorb them from food declines. So it's probably a good idea, and certainly can't hurt, to take a multivitamin-and-mineral pill after age fifty. And if you don't eat much fish, it might be wise to take a fish oil supplement too.

Eat more like the French. Or the Italians. Or the Japanese. Or the Indians. Or the Greeks. Confounding factors aside, people who eat according to the rules of a traditional food culture are generally much healthier than people eating a contemporary Western diet. This goes for the Japanese and other Asian diets as well as the traditional diets of Mexico, India, and the Mediterranean region, including France, Italy, and Greece. There may be exceptions to this rule — you do have to wonder about the Eastern European Jewish diet of my ancestors. Though who knows? Chicken and duck fat may turn out to be much healthier than scientists presently believe. (Weston Price certainly wouldn't be surprised.) I'm inclined to think any traditional diet will do; if it wasn't a healthy regimen, the diet and the people who followed it wouldn't still be around.

There are of course two dimensions to a traditional diet — the foods a culture eats and how they eat them — and both may be equally important to our health. Let's deal first with the content of traditional diets and save the form of it, or eating habits, for the next section.

In some respects, traditional diets resemble other vernacular creations of culture such as architecture. Through a long, incremental process of trial and error, cultures discover what works — how best to reconcile human needs with whatever nature has to offer us in a particular place. So the pitch of a roof reflects the amount of rain or snowfall in a particular region, growing steeper the greater the precipitation, and something like the spiciness of a cuisine reflects the local climate in another way. Eating spicy foods helps people keep cool; many spices also have antimicrobial properties, which is important in warm climates where food is apt to spoil rapidly. And indeed researchers have found that the hotter a climate is, the more spices will be found in the local cuisine.

Of course cuisines are not only concerned with health or even biology; many culinary practices are arbitrary and possibly even maladaptive, like the polishing of rice. Cuisines can have purely cultural functions; they're one of the ways a society expresses its identity and underscores its differences with other societies. (Religious food rules like kashruth or halal perform this function for, respectively, Jews and Muslims.) These cultural purposes might explain why cuisines tend to resist change; it is often said that the last place to look for signs of assimilation in an immigrant's home is the pantry. Though as food psychologist Paul Rozin points out, the abiding "flavor principles" of a cuisine — whether lemon and olive oil in the Mediterranean, soy sauce and ginger in Asia, or even ketchup in America — make it easier for a culture to incorporate useful new foods that might otherwise taste unacceptably foreign.

Yet more than many other cultural practices, eating is deeply rooted in nature — in human biology on one side and in the natural world on the other. The specific combinations of foods in a cuisine and the ways they are prepared constitute a deep reservoir of accumulated wisdom about diet and health and place. Many traditional culinary practices are the products of a kind of biocultural evolution, the ingenuity of which modern science occasionally figures out long after the fact. In Latin America, corn is traditionally eaten with beans; each plant is deficient in an essential amino acid that happens to be abundant in the other, so together corn and beans form a balanced diet in the absence of meat. Similarly, corn in these countries is traditionally ground or soaked with limestone, which makes available a B vitamin in the corn, the absence of which would otherwise lead to the deficiency disease called pellagra. Very often when a society adopts a new food without the food culture surrounding it, as happened when corn first came to Europe, Africa, and Asia, people get sick. The context in which a food is eaten can be nearly as important as the food itself.

The ancient Asian practice of fermenting soybeans and eating soy in the form of curds called tofu makes a healthy diet from a plant that eaten almost any other way would make people ill. The soybean itself is a notably inauspicious staple food; it contains a whole assortment of "antinutrients" — compounds that actually block the body's absorption of vitamins and minerals, interfere with the hormonal system, and prevent the body from breaking down the proteins in the soy itself. It took the food cultures of Asia to figure out how to turn this unpromising plant into a highly nutritious food. By boiling crushed soybeans in water to form a kind of milk and then precipitating the liquid by adding gypsum (calcium sulfate), cooks were able to form the soy into curds of highly digestible protein: tofu.

So how are these traditional methods of "food processing" different from newer kinds of food science? Only in that the traditional methods have stood the test of time, keeping people well nourished and healthy generation after generation. One of the hallmarks of a traditional diet is its essential conservatism. Traditions in food ways reflect long experience and often embody a nutritional logic that we shouldn't heedlessly overturn. So consider this subclause to the rule about eating a traditional diet:

Regard nontraditional foods with skepticism. Innovation is interesting, but when it comes to something like food, it pays to approach novelties with caution. If diets are the product of an evolutionary process, then a novel food or culinary innovation resembles a mutation: It *might* represent a revolutionary improvement, but it probably doesn't. It was really interesting when modernist architecture dispensed with the pitched roof; on the other hand, the flat roofs that replaced them tended to leak.

Soy again offers an interesting case in point. Americans are eating more soy products than ever before, thanks largely to the ingenuity of an industry eager to process and sell the vast amounts of subsidized soy coming off American and South American farms. But today we're eating soy in ways Asian cultures with much longer experience of the plant would not recognize: "Soy protein isolate," "soy isoflavones," "textured vegetable protein" from soy and soy oils (which now account for a fifth of the calories in the American diet) are finding their way into thousands of processed foods, with the result that Americans now eat more soy than the Japanese or the Chinese do.

Yet there are questions about the implications of these novel food products for our health. Soy isoflavones, found in most soy products, are compounds that resemble estrogen, and in fact bind to human estrogen receptors. But it is unclear whether these so-called phytoestrogens actually behave like estrogen in the body or only fool it into thinking they're estrogen. Either way the phytoestrogens might have an effect (good *or* bad) on the growth of certain cancers, the symptoms of menopause, and the function of the endocrine system. Because of these uncertainties, the FDA has declined to grant GRAS ("generally regarded as safe") status to soy isoflavones used as a food additive. As a senior scientist at the FDA's National Center for Toxicological Research wrote, "Confidence that soy products are safe is clearly based more on belief than hard data." Until those data come in, I feel more comfortable eating soy prepared in the traditional Asian style than according to novel recipes developed by processors like Archer Daniels Midland.

Don't look for the magic bullet in the traditional diet. In the same way that foods are more than the sum of their nutrient parts, dietary patterns seem to be more than the sum of the foods that comprise them. Oceans of ink have been spilled attempting to tease out and analyze the components of the Mediterranean diet, hoping to identify the X factor responsible for its healthfulness: Is it the olive oil? The fish? The wild greens? The garlic? The nuts? The French paradox too has been variously attributed to the salutary effects of red wine, olive oil, and even foie gras (liver is high in B vitamins and iron). Yet when researchers extract a single food from a diet of proven value, it usually fails to adequately explain why the people living on that diet live longer or have lower rates of heart disease or cancer than people eating a modern Western diet. The whole of a dietary pattern is evidently greater than the sum of its parts.

Some of these dietary parts flagrantly contradict current scientific thinking about healthy eating. By the standards of most official dietary guidelines, the French eat poorly: way too much saturated fat and wine. The Greeks too have their own paradox; defying the recommendation that we get no more than 30 percent of our calories from fats, they get 40 percent, most of it in the form of olive oil. So researchers begin looking for synergies between nutrients:

Might the antioxidants in the red wine help metabolize the fats? Perhaps. But it seems unlikely that any single food, nutrient, or mechanism will ever explain the French paradox; more likely, we will someday come to realize there never was a paradox. Dietary paradoxes are best thought of as breakdowns in nutritionist thinking, a sign of something wrong with the scientific consensus rather than the diet in question.

But the quest to pin down the X factor in the diets of healthy populations (PubMed, a scholarly index to scientific articles on medicine, lists 257 entries under "French Paradox" and another 828 under "Mediterranean Diet") goes on, because reductionist science is understandably curious and nutritionism demands it. If the secret ingredient could be identified, then processed foods could be reengineered to contain more of it, and we could go on eating much as before. The only way to profit from the wisdom of traditional diets (aside from writing books about them) is to break them down using reductionist science and then sell them for their nutrient parts.

In recent years a less reductive method of doing nutritional science has emerged, based on the idea of studying whole dietary patterns instead of individual foods or nutrients. The early results have tended to support the idea that traditional diets do indeed protect us from chronic disease and that these diets can be transferred from one place and population to another. Even some of the researchers associated with the Nurses' Health Study have begun doing dietary pattern analysis, in one case comparing a prudent diet modeled on Mediterranean and Asian patterns — high in fruits, vegetables, and fish and low in red meat and dairy products — with a typical Western diet featuring lots of meat (and processed meat), refined grains, sugary foods, french fries, and dairy products. (The study found "strong evidence" that the prudent dietary pattern may reduce the risk of coronary heart disease.)[*] Another recent study of a traditional plant-based diet found that even when you tested it against a low-fat Western diet that contained the same proportions of total fat, saturated fat, protein, carbohydrates, and cholesterol, the people on the traditional diet did much better by an important measure of cardiovascular health.

[*]Frank B. Hu, et al., "Prospective Study of Major Dietary Patterns and Risk of Coronary Heart Disease in Men," *American Journal of Clinical Nutrition,* 2000; 72:912–21.

What this suggests is that the addition of certain foods to the diet (Vegetables and fruits? Whole grains? Garlic?) may be more important than the subtraction of the usual nutritional suspects.[*]

*Christopher Gardner et al. "The Effect of a Plant-Based Diet on Plasma Lipids in Hypercholesterolemic Adults," *Annals of Internal Medicine,* 2005; 142: 725–33. Other similar trials have found striking protective effects in more traditional, plant-based dietary patterns that no single nutrient can adequately explain. In the D.A.S.H. (Dietary Approaches to Stop Hypertension) study, a diet rich in fruits and vegetables and low in saturated fat reduced blood pressure even when salt intake and weight remained unchanged. (Lawrence J. Appel, et al., "A Clinical Trial of the Effects of Dietary Patterns on Blood Pressure," *New England Journal of Medicine,* Vol. 336, No. 16, April 17, 1997.) Neither of these studies relied on food-frequency questionnaires; rather, the researchers prepared the meals for the participants. The Lyon Diet Heart Study found that the Mediterranean diet, when compared to a Western diet, offered protection against a second heart attack during the four years patients were followed. (Michel de Lorgeril et al., "Mediterranean Diet, Traditional Risk Factors, and the Rate of Cardiovascular Complications after Myocardial Infarc-

As the authors of the first study point out, the strength of such an approach is that "it more closely parallels the real world" in that "it can take into account complicated interactions among nutrients and non-nutrient substances in studies of free-living people." The weakness of such an approach is that "it cannot be specific about the particular nutrients responsible" for whatever health effects have been observed. Of course, this is a weakness only from the perspective of nutritionism. The inability to pin down the key nutrient matters much more to the scientist (and the food industry) than it does to us "free-living" eaters in the real world.

Have a glass of wine with dinner. Wine may not be the X factor in the French or Mediterranean diet, but it does seem to be an integral part of those dietary patterns. There is now abundant scientific evidence for the health benefits of alcohol to go with a few centuries of traditional belief and anecdotal evidence. Mindful of the social and health effects of alcoholism, public health authorities are loath to recommend drinking, but the fact is that people who drink moderately

tion," *Circulation,* 1999:99; 779–85.)

and regularly live longer and suffer considerably less heart disease than teetotalers.
Alcohol of any kind appears to reduce the
risk of heart disease, but the polyphenols in
red wine (resveratrol in particular) appear
to have unique protective qualities. The
benefits to your heart increase with the
amount of alcohol consumed up to about
four drinks a day (depending on your size),
yet drinking that much increases your risk
of dying from other causes (including
certain cancers and accidents), so most
experts recommend no more than two
drinks a day for men, one for women. The
health benefits of alcohol may depend as
much on the pattern of drinking as on the
amount: Drinking a little every day is better
than drinking a lot on the weekends, and
drinking with food is better than drinking
without it. (Food blunts some of the deleterious effects of alcohol by slowing its
absorption.) Also, a diet particularly rich in
plant foods, as the French and Mediterranean diets are, supplies precisely the B
vitamins that drinking alcohol depletes.
How fortunate! Someday science may comprehend all the complex synergies at work
in a traditional diet that includes wine, but
until then we can marvel at its accumulated
wisdom — and raise a glass to paradox.

FOUR:
NOT TOO MUCH: HOW TO EAT

If a food is more than the sum of its nutrients and a diet is more than the sum of its foods, it follows that a food culture is more than the sum of its menus — it embraces as well the set of manners, eating habits, and unspoken rules that together govern a people's relationship to food and eating. *How* a culture eats may have just as much of a bearing on health as *what* a culture eats. The foodstuffs of another people are often easier to borrow than their food habits, it's true, but to adopt some of these habits would do at least as much for our health and happiness as eaters.

What nutritionism sees when it looks at the French paradox is a lot of slender French people eating gobs of saturated fat washed down with wine. What it fails to see is a people with a completely different relationship to food than we have. Nutritionists pay far more attention to the chemistry of food than to the sociology or ecology of eating. All their studies of the benefits of red wine or foie gras overlook the fact that the French eat very differently than we do. They seldom snack, and they eat most of their food at meals shared with other people.

They eat small portions and don't come back for seconds. And they spend considerably more time eating than we do. Taken together, these habits contribute to a food culture in which the French consume fewer calories than we do, yet manage to enjoy them far more.

Paul Rozin has confirmed many of these observations in a comparison of French and American eating habits conducted in restaurants in Paris and Philadelphia. Rozin focused on portion size and time spent eating. He found that serving sizes in France, both in restaurants and supermarkets, are considerably smaller than they are in the United States. This matters because most people have what psychologists call a unit bias — we tend to believe that however big or small the portion served, that's the proper amount to eat. Rozin also found that the French spend considerably more time enjoying their tiny servings than we do our Brobdingnagian ones. "Although they eat less than Americans," Rozin writes, "the French spend more time eating, and hence get more food experience while eating less." He suggests that the French gift for extracting more food experience from fewer calories may help explain why the French are slimmer and healthier than we are. This sounds like an eminently sensible approach to eating and suggests an overarching policy that might nudge us in that direction.

Pay more, eat less. What the French case suggests is that there is a trade-off in eating between quantity and quality.

The American food system has for more than a century devoted its energies to quantity and price rather than to quality. Turning out vast quantities of so-so food sold in tremendous packages at a terrific price is what we do well. Yes, you can find exceptional food in America, and increasingly so, but historically the guiding principle has been, in the slogan of one supermarket chain, to "pile it high and sell it cheap."

There's no escaping the fact that better food — whether measured by taste or nutritional quality (which often correspond) — costs more, usually because it has been grown with more care and less intensively. Not everyone can afford to eat high-quality food in America, and that is shameful; however, those of us who can, should. Doing so benefits not only your health (by, among other things, reducing your exposure to pesticides and pharmaceuticals), but also the health of the people who grow the food as well as the people who live downstream and downwind of the farms where it is grown.

Another important benefit of paying more for better-quality food is that you're apt to eat less of it.

"Eat less" is the most unwelcome advice of all, but in fact the scientific case for eating a lot less than we presently do is compelling, whether or not you are overweight. Calorie restriction has repeatedly been shown to slow aging and prolong lifespan in animals, and some researchers believe it is the single strongest link between a change in the diet and the prevention of cancer. Put simply: Overeating promotes cell division, and promotes it most dramatically in cancer cells; cutting back on calories slows cell division. It also stifles the production of free radicals, curbs inflammation, and reduces the risk of most of the Western diseases.

"Eat less" is easier said than done, however, particularly in a culture of cheap and abundant calories with no deeply rooted set of rules to curb overeating. But other cultures do have such rules and we can try to emulate them. The French have their modest portions and taboo against seconds. The people of Okinawa, one of the longest-lived and healthiest populations in the world, practice a principle they call *hara ha-chi bu:* Eat until you are 80 percent full.

This is a sensible idea, but also easier said than done: How in the world do you know when you're 80 percent full? You'd need to be in closer touch with your senses than many Americans at the table have become. As Rozin and other psychologists have demonstrated, Americans typically eat not until they're full (and certainly not until they're 80 percent full) but rather until they receive some visual cue from their environment that it's time to stop: the bowl or package is empty, the plate is clean, or the TV show is over. Brian Wansink, a Cornell professor of marketing and nutritional science who has done several ingenious studies on portion size and appetite, concludes that Americans pay much more attention to external than to internal cues about satiety.[*]

[*]In one study Wansink rigged up bowls of soup in a restaurant so they would automatically refill from the bottom; those given the bottomless bowl ate 73 percent more soup than the subjects eating from an ordinary bowl; several ate as much as a quart. When one of these hearty eaters was asked his opinion of the soup, he said, "It's pretty good, and it's pretty filling." Indeed.

By comparison the French, who seem to attend more closely to all the sensual dimensions of eating, also pay more attention to the internal cues telling us we feel full.

So how might paying more for food help us eat less of it? In two ways. It is well established that how much we eat is strongly influenced by the cost of food in terms of both the money and effort required to put it on the table. The rise in obesity in America began around 1980, exactly when a flood of cheap calories started coming off American farms, prompted by the Nixon-era changes in agricultural policy. American farmers produced 600 more calories per person per day in 2000 than they did in 1980. But some calories got cheaper than others: Since 1980, the price of sweeteners and added fats (most of them derived, respectively, from subsidized corn and subsidized soybeans) dropped 20 percent, while the price of fresh fruits and vegetables increased by 40 percent. It is the cheaper and less healthful of these two kinds of calories on which Americans have been gorging.

These are precisely the kinds of calories found in convenience food — snacks, microwavable entrées, soft drinks, and packaged food of all kind — which happens to be the source of most of the 300 or so extra calories Americans have added to their daily diet since 1980. So these foods are cheap in a second sense too: They require very little, if any, time or effort to prepare, which is the other reason we eat more of them. How often would you eat french fries if you had to peel, wash, cut and fry them yourself — and then clean up the mess? Or ever eat Twinkies if you had to bake the little cakes and then squirt the filling into them and clean up?

Recently a group of Harvard economists seeking to advance an economic theory for the obesity epidemic correlated the rise in the average weight of Americans with a decline in the "time cost" of eating — cooking, cleaning up, and so on. They concluded that the widespread availability of cheap convenience foods could explain most of the twelve-pound increase in the weight of the average American since the early 1960s. They point out that in 1980 less than 10 percent of Americans owned a microwave; by 1999 that figure had reached 83 percent of households. As technology reduces the time cost of food, we tend to eat more of it.[*]

[*]David M. Cutler, et al., "Why Have Americans

My guess is that the converse still holds true, and that paying more for food — in every sense — will reduce the amount of it we eat. Several of the rules offered below are aimed in that direction. While it is true that many people simply can't afford to pay more for food, either in money or time or both, many more of us can. After all, just in the last decade or two we've somehow found the time in the day to spend several hours on the Internet and the money in the budget not only to pay for broadband service, but to cover a second phone bill and a new monthly bill for television, formerly free. For the majority of Americans, spending more for better food is less a matter of ability than priority. We spend a smaller percentage of our income on food than any other industrialized society; surely if we decided that the quality of our food mattered, we could afford to spend a few more dollars on it a week — and eat a little less of it.

Is it just a coincidence that as the portion of our income spent on food has declined, spending on health care has soared? In 1960

Become More Obese?," *Journal of Economic Perspectives,* Vol. 17, No. 3 (summer, 2003), pp. 93–118.

Americans spent 17.5 percent of their income on food and 5.2 percent of national income on health care. Since then, those numbers have flipped: Spending on food has fallen to 9.9 percent, while spending on health care has climbed to 16 percent of national income. I have to think that by spending a little more on healthier food we could reduce the amount we have to spend on health care.

To make the overall recommendation to "pay more, eat less" more palatable, consider that quality itself, besides tending to cost more, may have a direct bearing on the quantity you'll *want* to eat. The better the food, the less of it you need to eat in order to feel satisfied. All carrots are not created equal, and the best ones — the ones really worth savoring — are simply more satisfying, bite for bite. To borrow Paul Rozin's term, exceptional food offers us more "food experience" — per bite, per dish, per meal — and as the French have shown, you don't need a lot of food to have a rich food experience. Choose quality over quantity, food experience over mere calories.

Eat meals. This recommendation sounds almost as ridiculous as "eat food," but in America at least, it no longer goes without saying. We are snacking more and eating fewer meals together. Indeed, sociologists who study American eating habits no longer organize their results around the increasingly quaint concept of the meal: They now measure "eating occasions" and report that Americans have added to the traditional big three — breakfast, lunch, and dinner — an as-yet-untitled fourth daily eating occasion that lasts all day long: the constant sipping and snacking we do while watching TV, driving, and so on. One study found that among eighteen- to fifty-year-old Americans, roughly a fifth of all eating now takes place in the car.[*]

That one should feel the need to mount a defense of "the meal" is sad, but then I never would have thought "food" needed defending, either. Most readers will recall the benefits of eating meals without much prompting from me. It is at the dinner table that we socialize and civilize our children, teaching them manners and the art of conversation. At the dinner table parents can determine portion sizes, model eating

[*]The study, commissioned by industry and unpublished, was conducted by John Nihoff, a professor of gastronomy at the Culinary Institute of America.

and drinking behavior, and enforce social norms about greed and gluttony and waste. Shared meals are about much more than fueling bodies; they are uniquely human institutions where our species developed language and this thing we call culture. Do I need to go on?

All this is so well understood that when pollsters ask Americans if they eat together as a family most nights, they offer a resounding — and resoundingly untrue — reply in the affirmative. In fact, most American families today report eating dinner together three to four nights a week, but even those meals bear only the faintest resemblance to the Norman Rockwell ideal. If you install video cameras in the kitchen and dining-room ceilings above typical American families, as marketers for the major food companies have done, you'll quickly discover that the reality of the family dinner has diverged substantially from our image of it. Mom might still cook something for herself and sit at the table for a while, but she'll be alone for much of that time. That's because dad and each of the kids are likely to prepare an entirely different entrée for themselves, "preparing" in this case being a synonym for microwaving a package. Each family member might then join mom at the table for as long as it takes to eat, but not necessarily all at the same time. Technically, this kind of feeding counts as a family dinner in the survey results, though it's hard to believe it performs all the customary functions of a shared meal. Kraft or General Mills, for instance, is now determining the portion sizes, not mom, and the social value of sharing food is lost. It looks a lot more like a restaurant meal, where everyone orders his or her own dish. (Though the service isn't quite as good, because the entrées don't arrive at the same time.) Of course, people tend to eat more when they can have exactly what they want — which is precisely why the major food companies approve of this modernized family meal and have done everything in their considerable power to foster it. So they market different kinds of entrées to each member of the family (low carb for the dieting teenager, low cholesterol for dad, high fat for the eight-year-old, and so on), and engineer these "home meal replacements," as they're known in the trade, so that even the eight-year-old can safely microwave them.

But the biggest threat to the meal-as-we-knew-it is surely the snack, and snacking in recent years has colonized whole new parts of our day and places in our lives. Work, for example, used to be a more or less food-free stretch of time between meals, but no longer. Offices now typically have well-stocked kitchens, and it is apparently considered gauche at a business meeting or conference if a spread of bagels, muffins, pastries, and soft drinks is not provided at frequent intervals. Attending a recent conference on nutrition and health, of all things, I was astounded to see that in addition to the copious buffet at breakfast, lunch, and dinner, our hosts wheeled out a copious buffet halfway between breakfast and lunch and then again halfway between lunch and dinner, evidently worried that we would not be able to survive the long crossing from one meal to the next without a between-meal meal.

I may be showing my age, but didn't there used to be at least a mild social taboo against the between-meal snack? Well, it is gone. Americans today mark time all day long with nibbles of food and sips of soft drinks, which must be constantly at their sides, lest they expire during the haul between breakfast and lunch. (The snack food and beverage industry has surely been the great beneficiary of the new social taboo against smoking, which used to perform much the same time-marking function.) We have reengineered our cars to accommodate our snacks, adding bigger cup holders and even refrigerated glove compartments, and we've reengineered foods to be more easily eaten in the car. According to the Harvard economists' calculations, the bulk of the calories we've added to our diet over the past twenty years has come in the form of snacks. I don't need to point out that these snacks tend not to consist of fruits and vegetables. (Not even at my nutrition conference.) Or that the portion sizes have swelled or that the snacks themselves consist mainly of cleverly flavored and configured arrangements of refined carbohydrates, hydrogenated oils, corn sweeteners, and salt.

To counter the rise of the snack and restore the meal to its rightful place, consider as a start these few rules of thumb:

Do all your eating at a table. No, a desk is not a table.

Don't get your fuel from the same place your car does. American gas stations now make more money selling food (and cigarettes) than gasoline, but consider what kind of food this is: except perhaps for the milk and water, it's all highly processed

nonperishable snack foods and extravagantly sweetened soft drinks in hefty twenty-
ounce bottles. Gas stations have become
processed-corn stations: ethanol outside for
your car and high-fructose corn syrup inside
for you.

Try not to eat alone. Americans are increasingly eating in solitude. Though there is
research suggesting that light eaters will eat
more when they dine with others (probably
because they spend more time at the table),
for people prone to overeating, communal
meals tend to limit consumption, if only
because we're less likely to stuff ourselves
when others are watching. This is precisely
why so much food marketing is designed to
encourage us to eat in front of the TV or in
the car: When we eat mindlessly and alone,
we eat more. But regulating appetite is the
least of it: The shared meal elevates eating
from a mechanical process of fueling the
body to a ritual of family and community,
from mere animal biology to an act of
culture.

Consult your gut. As the psychologists have
demonstrated, most of us allow external,
and mostly visual, cues to determine how
much we eat. The larger the portion, the

more we eat; the bigger the container, the more we pour; the more conspicuous the vending machine, the more we buy from it; the closer the bowl of M&Ms, the more of them we eat. All of which makes us easy marks for food marketers eager to sell us yet more food.

As in so many areas of modern life, the culture of food has become a culture of the eye. But when it comes to eating, it pays to cultivate the other senses, which often provide more useful and accurate information. Does this peach smell as good as it looks? Does the third bite of that dessert taste anywhere near as good as the first? I could certainly eat more of this, but am I really still hungry?

Supposedly it takes twenty minutes before the brain gets the word that the belly is full; unfortunately most of us take considerably less than twenty minutes to finish a meal, with the result that the sensation of feeling full exerts little if any influence on how much we eat. What this suggests is that eating more slowly, and then consulting our sense of satiety, might help us to eat less. The French are better at this than we are, as Brian Wansink discovered when he asked a group of French people how they knew when to stop eating. "When I feel full," they replied. (What a novel idea! The Americans said things like "When my plate is clean" or "When I run out.") Perhaps it is their long, leisurely meals that give the French the opportunity to realize when they're full.

At least until we learn to eat more slowly and attend more closely to the information of our senses, it might help to work on altering the external clues we rely on in eating on the theory that it's probably better to manipulate ourselves than to allow marketers to manipulate us. Wansink offers dozens of helpful tips in a recent book called *Mindless Eating: Why We Eat More Than We Think,* though I warn you they're all vaguely insulting to your sense of yourself as a creature in possession of free will.

Serve smaller portions on smaller plates; serve food and beverages from small containers (even if this means repackaging things bought in jumbo sizes); leave detritus on the table — empty bottles, bones, and so forth — so you can see how much you've eaten or drunk; use glasses that are more vertical than horizontal (people tend to pour more into squat glasses); leave healthy foods in view, unhealthy ones out of view; leave serving bowls in the kitchen rather than on the table to discourage second helpings.

Eat slowly. Not just so you'll be more likely to know when to stop. I mean "slow" in the sense of deliberate and knowledgeable eating promoted by Slow Food, the Italian-born movement dedicated to the principle that "a firm defense of quiet material pleasure is the only way to oppose the universal folly of Fast Life." The organization, which was founded in response to the arrival of American fast food in Rome during the 1980s, seeks to reacquaint (or in some cases acquaint) people with the satisfactions of well-grown and well-prepared food enjoyed at leisurely communal meals. It sounds like an elitist club for foodies (which, alas, it sometimes can be), but at its most thoughtful, Slow Food offers a coherent protest against, and alternative to, the Western diet and way of eating, indeed to the whole ever-more-desperate Western way of life. Slow Food aims to elevate quality over quantity and believes that doing so depends on cultivating our sense of taste as well as rebuilding the relationships between producers and consumers that the industrialization of our food has destroyed. "Food quality depends on consumers who respect the work of farmers and are willing to educate their senses," Carlo Petrini, Slow Food's founder, has said. When that happens, "they become precious allies for producers." Even connoisseurship can have a politics, as when it deepens our appreciation for the work of the people who produce our food and ruins our taste for the superficial pleasures of fast food.

It is no accident that Slow Food has its roots in Italy, a country much less enamored of the "folly of Fast Life" than the United States, and you have to wonder whether it's realistic to think the American way of eating can be reformed without also reforming the whole American way of life. Fast food is precisely the way you'd expect a people to eat who put success at the center of life, who work long hours (with two careers per household), get only a couple of weeks vacation each year, and who can't depend on a social safety net to cushion them from life's blows. But Slow Food's wager is that making time and slowing down to eat, an activity that happens three times a day and ramifies all through a culture, is precisely the wedge that can begin to crack the whole edifice.

To eat slowly, in the Slow Food sense, is to eat with a fuller knowledge of all that is involved in bringing food out of the earth and to the table. Undeniably, there are pleasures to be had eating that are based on the opposite — on knowing precious little; indeed, they sometimes depend on it. The fast-food hamburger has been brilliantly engineered to offer a succulent and tasty first bite, a bite that in fact would be impossible to enjoy if the eater could accurately picture the feedlot and the slaughterhouse and the workers behind it or knew anything about the "artificial grill flavor" that made that first bite so convincing. This is a hamburger to hurry through, no question. By comparison, eating a grass-fed burger when you can picture the green pastures in which the animal grazed is a pleasure of another order, not a simple one, to be sure, but one based on knowledge rather than ignorance and gratitude rather than indifference.

To eat slowly, then, also means to eat deliberately, in the original sense of that word: "from freedom" instead of compulsion. Many food cultures, particularly those at less of a remove from the land than ours, have rituals to encourage this sort of eating, such as offering a blessing over the food or saying grace before the meal. The point, it seems to me, is to make sure that we don't eat thoughtlessly or hurriedly, and that knowledge and gratitude will inflect our pleasure at the table. I don't ordinarily offer any special words before a meal, but I do sometimes recall a couple of sentences written by Wendell Berry, which do a good job of getting me to eat more deliberately:

Eating with the fullest pleasure — pleasure, that is, that does not depend on ignorance — is perhaps the profoundest enactment of our connection with the world. In this pleasure we experience and celebrate our dependence and our gratitude, for we are living from mystery, from creatures we did not make and powers we cannot comprehend.

Words such as these are one good way to foster a more deliberate kind of eating, but perhaps an even better way (as Berry himself has suggested) is for eaters to involve themselves in food production to whatever extent they can, even if that only means planting a few herbs on a sunny windowsill or foraging for edible greens and wild mushrooms in the park. If much of our carelessness in eating owes to the ease with which the industrial eater can simply forget all that is at stake, both for himself and for the world, then getting reacquainted with how food is grown and prepared can provide a useful reminder. So one last rule:

Cook and, if you can, plant a garden. To take part in the intricate and endlessly interesting processes of providing for our sustenance is the surest way to escape the culture of fast food and the values implicit in it: that food should be fast, cheap, and easy; that food is a product of industry, not nature; that food is fuel, and not a form of communion, with other people as well as with other species — with nature.

So far I am more at home in the garden than the kitchen, though I can appreciate how time spent in either place alters one's relationship to food and eating. The garden offers a great many solutions, practical as well as philosophical, to the whole problem of eating well. My own vegetable garden is modest in scale — a densely planted patch in the front yard only about twenty feet by ten — but it yields an astonishing cornucopia of produce, so much so that during the summer months we discontinue our CSA box and buy little but fruit from the farmers' market. And though we live on a postage-stamp city lot, there's room enough for a couple of fruit trees too: a lemon, a fig, and a persimmon. To the problem of being able to afford high-quality organic produce the garden offers the most straightforward solution: The food you grow yourself is fresher than any you can buy, and it costs nothing but an hour or two of work each week plus the price of a few packets of seed.

The work of growing food contributes to your health long before you sit down to eat it, of course, but there is something particularly fitting about enlisting your body in its own sustenance. Much of what we call recreation or exercise consists of pointless physical labor, so it is especially satisfying when we can give that labor a point. But gardening consists of mental work as well: learning about the different varieties; figuring out which do best under the conditions of your garden; acquainting yourself with the various microclimates — the subtle differences in light, moisture, and soil quality across even the tiniest patch of earth; and devising ways to outwit pests without resorting to chemicals. None of this work is terribly difficult; much of it is endlessly gratifying, and never more so than in the hour immediately before dinner, when I take a knife and a basket out to the garden to harvest whatever has declared itself ripest and tastiest.

Among other things, tending a garden reminds us of our ancient evolutionary bargain with these ingenious domestic species — how cleverly they insinuate themselves into our lives, repaying the care and space we give them with the gift of good food. Each has its own way of announcing — through a change of color, shape, smell, texture, or taste — that the moment when it has the very most to offer us, when it is at its sweetest and most nourishing, has arrived: *Pick me!*

Not that everything in the garden always works out so well; it doesn't, but there is a value in the inevitable failures too. Whenever your produce is anything less than gorgeous and delicious, gardening cultivates in you a deep respect for the skill of the farmer who knows how consistently to get it right.

When the basket of produce lands on the kitchen counter, when we start in on the cleaning and cutting and chopping, we're thinking about a dozen different things — what to make, how to make it — but nutrition, or even health, is probably not high on the list. Look at this food. There are no ingredients labels, no health claims, nothing to read except maybe a recipe. It's hard when contemplating such produce to think in terms of nutrients or chemical compounds; no, this is food, so fresh it's still alive, communicating with us by scent and color and taste. The good cook takes in all this sensory information and only then decides what to do with the basket of possibilities on the counter: what to combine it with; how, and how much, to "process" it. Now the culture of the kitchen takes over. That culture is embodied in those enduring traditions we call cuisines, any one of which contains more wisdom about diet and health than you will find in any nutrition journal or journalism. The cook does not need to know, as the scientists have recently informed us, that cooking the tomatoes with olive oil makes the lycopene in them more available to our bodies. No, the cook already knew that olive oil with tomatoes is a really good idea.

As cook in your kitchen you enjoy an omniscience about your food that no amount of supermarket study or label reading could hope to match. Having retaken control of the meal from the food scientists and processors, you know exactly what is and is not in it: There are no questions about high-fructose corn syrup, or ethoxylated diglycerides, or partially hydrogenated soy oil, for the simple reason that you didn't ethoxylate or partially hydrogenate anything, nor did you add any additives. (Unless, that is, you're the kind of cook who starts with a can of Campbell's cream of mushroom soup, in which case all bets are off.) To reclaim this much control over one's food, to take it back from industry and science, is no small thing; indeed, in our time cooking from scratch and growing any of your own food qualify as subversive acts.

And what these acts subvert is nutritionism: the belief that food is foremost about nutrition and nutrition is so complex that only experts and industry can possibly supply it. When you're cooking with food as alive as this — these gorgeous and semigorgeous fruits and leaves and flesh — you're in no danger of mistaking it for a commodity, or a fuel, or a collection of chemical nutrients. No, in the eye of the cook or the gardener or the farmer who grew it, this food reveals itself for what it is: no mere *thing* but a web of relationships among a great many living beings, some of them human, some not, but each of them dependent on the other, and all of them ultimately rooted in soil and nourished by sunlight. I'm thinking of the relationship between the plants and the soil, between the grower and the plants and animals he or she tends, between the cook and the growers who supply the ingredients, and between the cook and the people who will soon come to the table to enjoy the meal. It is a large community to nourish and be nourished by. The cook in the kitchen preparing a meal from plants and animals at the end of this shortest of food chains has a great many things to worry about, but "health" is simply not one of them, because it is given.

ACKNOWLEDGMENTS

I've dedicated *In Defense of Food* to two editors, Ann Godoff and Gerry Marzorati, because the book would not exist without them. It began with an assignment from Gerry, who, over lunch one afternoon at a restaurant in Oakland, proposed that I learn all that I could about diet and health and then write an essay about it. When that essay was published in *The New York Times Magazine* a year ago, under the title "Unhappy Meals," Ann Godoff, my longtime book editor, telephoned to suggest the piece might hold the germ of a book — this book. I mention all this because I suspect many readers assume books spring full blown from the heads of writers, when in fact many of them spring, half baked, from the heads of brilliant editors. I'm unusually fortunate to have two of the very best ones deciding how I should spend my time. I'm doubly fortunate that Ann and Gerry also

279

happen to be two of my dearest friends. Heartfelt thanks to both of you.

Ann and Gerry weren't the only editors who had a hand in this book, though the others don't wear the title or receive compensation for their labors (beyond this paragraph). As with every one of my books, Judith Belzer read the manuscript more times than anyone should have to and improved it in countless ways. I can no longer even imagine what it would be like to write a book without her as my first reader, and you can have no idea just how many lame sentences and lousy ideas she has kept out of print. As in the past, Mark Edmundson and Michael Schwarz also read the book in manuscript and made priceless suggestions; I couldn't have more supportive or stimulating colleagues. Thanks too to Jack Hitt, who's read all my books in galleys and helped me to figure out what I've written — not always so obvious. Christopher Gardner, a nutrition scientist at Stanford University School of Medicine, reviewed the manuscript for scientific accuracy and rescued me from numerous errors of fact and interpretation; of course any that remain are mine alone. His own pioneering research in dietary patterns was also very helpful in developing my recommendations in part three.

I owe an incalculable debt of gratitude to Adrienne Davich, a gifted journalist (and former student) who did a splendid and heroic job of researching the book and fact-checking the manuscript. Adrienne immersed herself in the medical literature, scoured the Berkeley library and databases for information, and worked the phone confirming facts right up to press time. I don't exaggerate when I say this book might still not be finished if not for her zeal, intelligence, scrupulousness, judgment, and unfailing good humor in the face of a daunting deadline. I also want to thank my assistant Jaime Gross, for her indispensable help and constant good cheer, as well as my past and present students at the Graduate School of Journalism, who contribute more to my work than they probably realize.

This book is in many ways a work of synthesis, built on a foundation of research and thinking laid by others. In educating myself on the subject of food, health, and agriculture over the past several years, I've been fortunate to have four of the wisest and most generous teachers: Joan Gussow, Marion Nestle, Alice Waters, and Wendell Berry — you are abiding inspirations. For their insights and information in conversations and e-mail exchanges, I'm also pleased to be able to acknowledge and thank: Susan Allport, Gyorgy Scrinis (coiner of the term *nutritionism*), Walter Willett, Joseph Hibbeln, Gladys Block, Geoffrey Cannon, Andrew Weil, Gary Nabhan, Bill Lands, David Ludwig, Jim Kaput, Alyson Mitchell, Brian Halweil, Bruce Ames, Martin Renner, and Kerin O'Dea. I hope I've done justice to your work. Much of what I know about agriculture and food systems I learned from Joel Salatin and George Naylor; and about eating well from Carlo Petrini, Angelo Garro, Dan Barber, everyone at Chez Panisse, and of course my mother, Corky Pollan. The growers in my own local food chain have also contributed much to my thinking about food and health: Thanks to Judith Redmond and everyone else at Full Belly Farm (my CSA), David Evans at Marin Sun Farms, and all the farmers at the Thursday farmers' market in Berkeley.

Alex Star, my story editor at *The New York Times Magazine,* helped to focus my thinking in a series of conversations; his gentle but persistent prodding kept the project on track, and his incisive questions helped sharpen my arguments. I'm also grateful to the hundreds of readers who e-mailed me after the publication of both *The Omnivore's*

Dilemma and "Unhappy Meals," offering invaluable criticisms, leads, reading suggestions, and provocations; this book is much better for your contributions.

At The Penguin Press, I get to work with not only the most talented but also the *nicest* people in book publishing: Tracy Locke, Sarah Hutson, Liza Darnton, Lindsay Whalen, Maggie Sivon, and Jacqueline Fischetti. Publishing a book is seldom thought of as a pleasant process, but at Penguin these days it actually almost is. I count on Amanda Urban, my literary agent for the past twenty years, for sage and completely unvarnished advice, and once again she delivered the goods. Binky is almost never wrong about anything. Though I would like to take this opportunity to remind her that, when I left New England for laid-back California, she predicted I would never complete another book. Here's number two.

I owe a debt to three very special institutions for making that possible and supporting the writing of this book: the Graduate School of Journalism at Berkeley, where I've taught since 2003 (thank you, Orville Schell and colleagues); the John S. and James L. Knight Foundation, which has supported my research since I came to Berkeley (thank you, Eric Newton); and Mesa Refuge, for lending me the cabin overlooking Tomales Bay where I wrote the first pages of this book under nearly ideal circumstances (thank you, Peter Barnes).

Finally to Isaac, kitchen collaborator, supertaster, fast friend of the carbohydrate, thank you for all the wonderful ideas and suggestions, even for coining the word "cornography" to describe your father's work. The prize of you and your mother's company at the dinner table at the end of the day is what makes the writing possible.

SOURCES

Listed below, by section, are the principal works referred to in the text as well as others that supplied me with facts or contributed to my thinking. Web site URLs are current as of September 2007. All cited articles by me are available at www.michaelpollan .com.

Introduction: An Eater's Manifesto

Glassner, Barry. *The Gospel of Food* (New York: HarperCollins Publishers, 2007).

Kantrowitz, Barbara, and Claudia Kalb. "Food News Blues." *Newsweek* (March 13, 2006).

Kass, Leon. *The Hungry Soul* (New York: The Free Press, 1994).

Mozaffarian, Dariush, and Eric B. Rimm. "Fish Intake, Contaminants, and Human Health: Evaluating the Risks and the Benefits." *Journal of the American Medical Association.* 296.15 (2006):1885–99.

Nesheim, Malden C., et al. "Seafood Choices: Balancing Benefits and Risks" (Washington, D.C.: National Academies Press, 2006).

Nestle, Marion. *Food Politics* (Berkeley: University of California Press, 2002).

Pollan, Michael. *The Omnivore's Dilemma* (New York: The Penguin Press, 2006).

————. "Our National Eating Disorder." *New York Times Magazine,* (October 17, 2004).

Prentice, Ross L. "Low-Fat Dietary Pattern and Risk of Invasive Breast Cancer: The Women's Health Initiative Randomized Controlled Dietary Modification Trial." *Journal of the American Medical Association.* 295.6 (2006): 629–42.

Roberts, Paul. "The New Food Anxiety." *Psychology Today* (March/April, 1998).

Rozin, Paul. "The Selection of Foods by Rats, Humans, and Other Animals" in *Advances in the Study of Behavior,* Vol. 6. Edited by J. Rosenblatt, R. A. Hilde, C. Beer, and E. Shaw (New York: Academic Press, 1976), pp. 21–76. The phrase "the omnivore's dilemma" is usually credited to Rozin, who studies the psychology of food choices.

Scrinis, Gyorgy. "Sorry Marge." *Meanjin.* 61.4 (2002): 108–16. Scrinis coined the term "nutritionism" in this illuminating article.

Temple, Norman J., and Denis P. Burkitt. *Western Diseases* (New Jersey: Humana Press Inc., 1994).

Trivedi, Bijal. "The Good, the Fad, and the Unhealthy." *New Scientist* (September 23, 2006).

Part One: The Age of Nutritionism

On the history of nutrition science and the evolution of dietary advice:

Brock, William H. *Justus von Liebig: The Chemical Gatekeeper* (Cambridge: Cambridge University Press, 1997).

Cambridge World History of Food, The: Volume One, edited by Kenneth F. Kiple and Kriemhild Conee Ornelas (Cambridge: Cambridge University Press, 2000).

Ibid.: *Volume Two,* edited by Kenneth F. Kiple and Kriemhild Conee Ornelas (Cambridge: Cambridge University Press, 2000).

Cannon, Geoffrey. *The Fate of Nations: Food and Nutrition Policy in the New World.* The Caroline Walker Lecture 2003, given at the Royal Society (London: Caroline Walker Trust, 2003). Can be obtained online at www.cwt.org.uk.

————. "Nutrition: The New World Map." *Asia Pacific Journal of Clinical Nutrition*. 11 (2002): S480–S97.

"Effect of Vitamin E and Beta Carotene on the Incidence of Lung Cancer and Other Cancers in Male Smokers, The. The Alpha-Tocopherol, Beta Carotene Cancer Prevention Study Group." *New England Journal of Medicine*. 330.15 (1994): 1029–35.

Freudenheim, Jo L. "Study Design and Hypothesis Testing: Issues in the Evaluation of Evidence from Research in Nutritional Epidemiology." *American Journal of Clinical Nutrition*. 69 (1999): 1315S–21S.

Glassner, Barry. *The Gospel of Food* (New York: HarperCollins Publishers, 2007).

Kantrowitz, Barbara, and Claudia Kalb. "Food News Blues." *Newsweek* (March 13, 2006).

Levenstein, Harvey. *Paradox of Plenty* (Berkeley: University of California Press, 2003).

————. *Revolution at the Table: The Transformation of the American Diet* (Berkeley: University of California Press, 2003). Includes an excellent account of food faddism in America.

Melton, Lisa. "The Antioxidant Myth." *New*

Scientist (August 5–11, 2006).

Planck, Nina. *Real Food: What to Eat and Why* (New York: Bloomsbury, 2006).

Scrinis, Gyorgy. "Sorry Marge." *Meanjin.* 61.4 (2002): 108–16.

Shapiro, Laura. *Perfection Salad: Women and Cooking at the Turn of the Century* (New York: Random House, 2001).

Taubes, Gary. *Good Calories, Bad Calories* (New York: Knopf, 2007).

———. "The Soft Science of Dietary Fat." *Science.* 291.30 (March 2001).

———. "What if It's All Been a Big Fat Lie?" *New York Times* (July 7, 2002).

Trivedi, Bijal. "The Good, the Fad, and the Unhealthy." *New Scientist* (September 23, 2006).

U.S. Department of Health and Human Services. *The Surgeon General's Report on Nutrition and Health* (Washington, D.C., 1988).

U.S. Senate Select Committee on Nutrition and Human Needs. *Dietary Goals for the United States* (Washington, D.C., 1977).

On the contemporary food environment and food marketing:

Hartman, Harvey, and Jarrett Paschel.

"Understanding Obesity: Practical Suggestions for the Obesity Crisis" (Bellevue: The Hartman Group, Inc., 2006). Interesting anthropological analysis of how American eating habits contribute to obesity.

Lofstock, John. "Boosting Impulse Sales at the Checkout Counter." *Convenience Store Decisions* (January 11, 2006).

Martin, Andrew. "Makers of Sodas Try a New Pitch: They're Healthy." *New York Times* (March 7, 2007).

Merill, Richard A., et al. "Like Mother Used to Make: An Analysis of FDA Standards of Identity." *Columbia Law Review.* 74.4 (May 1974). Contains a good account of the FDA's 1973 decision to repeal its imitation rule.

Nestle, Marion. *Food Politics* (Berkeley: University of California Press, 2002).

———. *What to Eat* (New York: North Point Press, 2006).

Simon, Michele. *Appetite for Profit* (New York: Nation Books, 2006).

On the controversies surrounding modern nutrition science and its methods, the literature is endless. A good place to start appreciating the complexities, if not impossibilities, of the field is Marion Nestle's excellent epilogue to *Food Politics*. Gary Taubes offers a thorough critique of both epidemiological and clinical nutrition research in *Good Calories, Bad Calories*. For more on the methodology of nutrition science:

Belanger, C.F., C.H. Hennekens, B. Rosner et al. "The Nurses' Health Study." *American Journal of Nursing.* (1978): 1039–40.

Campbell, T. Colin. "Letters to the Editor: Animal Protein and Ischemic Heart Disease." *American Journal of Clinical Nutrition.* 71.3 (2000): 849–50.

Freudenheim, Jo L. "Study Design and Hypothesis Testing: Issues in the Evaluation of Evidence from Research in Nutritional Epidemiology." *American Journal of Clinical Nutrition.* 69 suppl (1999): 1315S–21S.

Giovannucci, Edward, et al. "A Comparison of Prospective and Retrospective Assessments of Diet in the Study of Breast Cancer." *American Journal of Epidemiology.* 137.5 (1993): 502–11.

Horner, Neilann K. "Participant Characteristics Associated with Errors in Self-Reported Energy Intake from the Women's Health Initiative Food-Frequency Questionnaire." *American Journal of Clinical Nutrition*. 76 (2002): 766–73.

Hu, Frank B., and Walter Willett. "Letters to the Editor: Reply to TC Campbell." *American Journal of Clinical Nutrition*. 71.3 (2000): 850–51.

Hu, Frank B., et al. "Reproducibility and Validity of Dietary Patterns Assessed with a Food-Frequency Questionnaire." *American Journal of Clinical Nutrition*. 69 (1999): 243–49.

Kristal, Alan R., et al. "Is It Time to Abandon the Food Frequency Questionnaire?" *Cancer Epidemiology Biomarkers Prevention*. 14.12 (2005): 2826–28.

Liu, Simin, et al. "Fruit and Vegetable Intake and Risk of Cardiovascular Disease: The Women's Health Study." *American Journal of Clinical Nutrition*. 72 (2000): 922–28.

Napoli, Maryann. "Prevention Advice to Women Doesn't Hold Up." Center for Medical Consumers Web site (March 2006). Available online at www.medical consumers.org.

Ostrzenski, Adam, and Katarzyna M. Ostrzenska. "WHI Clinical Trial Revisit: Imprecise Scientific Methodology Disqualifies the Study's Outcomes." *American*

Journal of Obstetrics and Gynecology. 193 (2005): 1599–1604.

Rosner, B., W. C. Willett, et al. "Correction of Logistic Regression Relative Risk Estimates and Confidence Intervals for Systematic Within-Person Measurement Error." *Statistics in Medicine.* 8 (1989): 1051–69.

Stein, Karen. "After the Media Feeding Frenzy: Whither the Women's Health Initiative Dietary Modification Trial?" *Journal of the American Dietetic Association.* (2006): 794–800.

Taubes, Gary. "Epidemiology Faces Its Limits." *Science.* 269.5221 (1995): 164–69.

———. *Good Calories, Bad Calories* (New York: Knopf, 2007).

Twombly, Renee. "Negative Women's Health Initiative Findings Stir Consternation, Debate Among Researchers." *Journal of the National Cancer Institute.* 98.8 (April 19, 2006).

Willett, Walter C. "Invited Commentary: A Further Look at Dietary Questionnaire Validation." *American Journal of Epidemiology.* 154.12 (2001): 1100–1102.

———, and Frank B. Hu. "Not the Time to Abandon the Food Frequency Questionnaire: Point." *Cancer Epidemiology Biomarkers Prevention.* 15.10 (2006): 1757–58.

On the subject of dietary fat and health:

Beresford, Shirley A. "Low-Fat Dietary Pattern and Risk of Colorectal Cancer: The Women's Health Initiative Randomized Controlled Dietary Modification Trial." *Journal of the American Medical Association.* 295.6 (2006): 643–654.

Dietary Fats and Health. Edited by E. G. Perkins and W. J. Visek (Champaign, IL: American Oil Chemists' Society, 1983). This book includes (from the Harshaw Chemical Company) Robert C. Hastert's article "Hydrogenation — A Tool, Not an Epithet," on pages 53–69.

Enig, Mary G. *Know Your Fats: The Complete Primer for Understanding the Nutrition of Fats, Oils, and Cholesterol* (Silver Spring, MD: Bethesda Press, 2000). Enig is hardly mainstream, but she was one of the first scientists to raise questions about the lipid hypothesis and sound the alarm about trans fats.

——, and Sally Fallon. "The Oiling of America" (The Weston A. Price Foundation, 2000). Available online at http://

www.westonaprice.org/knowyourfats/
oiling.html.

Howard, Barbara V., et al. "Low-Fat Dietary
Pattern and Risk of Cardiovascular Disease: The Women's Health Initiative Randomized Controlled Dietary Modification
Trial." *Journal of the American Medical Association*. 295.6 (2006): 655–66.

Hu, Frank B., et al. "Types of Dietary Fat
and Risk of Coronary Heart Disease: A
Critical Review." *Journal of the American
College of Nutrition*. 20.1 (2001): 5–19.

Ludwig, David S. "Clinical Update: The
Low-Glycemic-Index Diet." *The Lancet*.
369.9565 (2007): 890–92.

Prentice, Ross L. "Low-Fat Dietary Pattern
and Risk of Invasive Breast Cancer: The
Women's Health Initiative Randomized
Controlled Dietary Modification Trial."
*Journal of the American Medical Associa-
tion*. 295.6 (2006): 629–42.

Taubes, Gary. *Good Calories, Bad Calories*
(New York: Knopf, 2007). Taubes's reporting on and analysis of the lipid hypothesis
is groundbreaking.

———. "The Soft Science of Dietary Fat."
Science. 291.30 (March 2001).

———. "What if It's All Been a Big Fat
Lie?" *New York Times Magazine* (July 7,
2002). This article almost single-handedly

launched the second Atkins craze and the great carbophobia of 2002–2003.

On the links between diet and diseases:

Campbell, T. Colin, and Thomas M. Campbell II. *The China Study* (Dallas: BenBella Books, Inc., 2006).

Ford, Earl S., et al. "Explaining the Decrease in U.S. Deaths from Coronary Disease, 1980–2000." *New England Journal of Medicine.* 356.23 (2007): 2388–98.

Key, Timothy J., et al. "Diet, Nutrition and the Prevention of Cancer." *Public Health Nutrition.* 7.1A (2004): 187–200.

National Research Council. *Diet, Nutrition and Cancer* (Washington, D.C.: National Academy Press, 1982).

Nestle, Marion. *Food Politics* (Berkeley: University of California Press, 2002).

Nutritional Genomics: Discovering the Path to Personalized Nutrition. Edited by Jim Kaput and Raymond L. Rodriguez (Hoboken, NJ: John Wiley & Sons, Inc., 2006). This volume includes Walter Willett's article "The Pursuit of Optimal Diets: A Progress Report."

Nutritional Health: Strategies for Disease Prevention. Edited by Ted Wilson and Norman J. Temple (Totowa, NJ: Humana Press, Inc., 2001).

Rosamond, Wayne D., et al. "Trends in the Incidence of Myocardial Infarction and in Mortality Due to Coronary Heart Disease, 1987 to 1994." *New England Journal of Medicine.* 339.13 (1998): 861–67.

Willett, Walter C. "Diet and Cancer: One View at the Start of the Millennium." *Cancer Epidemiology, Biomarkers & Prevention.* 10 (2001): 3–8.

———. "Diet and Health: What Should We Eat?" *Science.* 264.5158 (1994): 532–37.

———. *Eat, Drink, and Be Healthy: The Harvard Medical School Guide to Healthy Eating* (New York: Free Press, 2001).

World Cancer Research Fund. *Food, Nutrition and the Prevention of Cancer: A Global Perspective.* (Washington, D.C.: American Institute for Cancer Research, 1997).

On nutritionism and its social and psychological effects:

Roberts, Paul. "The New Food Anxiety." *Psychology Today.* (March/April, 1998).

Rozin, Paul, et al. "Food and Life, Pleasure and Worry, Among American College Students: Gender Differences and Regional Similarities." *Journal of Personality and Social Psychology.* 85.1 (2003): 132–41.

Rozin, Paul. "Human Food Intake and Choice: Biological, Psychological and Cultural Perspectives." (Philadelphia: University of Pennsylvania, 2002). Available online at http://www.danone-institute.com/publications/book/pdf/food__selection__01__rozin.pdf.

———, et al. "Lay American Conceptions of Nutrition: Dose Insensitivity, Categorical Thinking, Contagion, and the Monotonic Mind." *Health Psychology.* 15.6 (1996): 438–47.

———, et al. "The Ecology of Eating: Smaller Portion Sizes in France Than in the United States Help Explain the French Paradox." *Psychological Science.* 14.5 (2003): 450–54.

Scrinis, Gyorgy, and Rosemary Stanton. "A Diet Thin on Science." *The Age* (August 29, 2005).

Scrinis, Gyorgy. "Engineering the Food Chain." *Arena Magazine.* 77 (2005): 37–39.

———. "High in Protein, Low in Fat and Too Good to Be True." *Sydney Morning Herald* (April 7, 2006).

———. "Labels: An Unhealthy Trend." *The*

Age (December 30, 2005).

———. "Sorry Marge." *Meanjin.* 61.4 (2002): 108–16.

Part Two: The Western Diet and the Diseases of Civilization

On the Western diet and its links to the Western diseases:

Diamond, Jared. *Guns, Germs, and Steel* (New York: W. W. Norton & Company, 1999).

Diet of Man: Needs and Wants. Edited by John Yudkin (London: Applied Science Publishers Ltd., 1978).

Drummond, J.C., and Anne Wilbraham. *The Englishman's Food: A History of Five Centuries of English Diet* (Oxford: Alden Press, 1939).

Milburn, Michael P. "Indigenous Nutrition." *American Indian Quarterly.* 28.3 (2004): 411–34.

Nabhan, Gary Paul. *Why Some Like It Hot: Food, Genes, and Cultural Diversity* (Washington, D.C.: Island Press, 2004).

Northbourne, Christopher James (5th Lord Northbourne). *Look to the Land* (London: J. M. Dent & Sons, 1940). New edition: (Hillsdale, NY: Sophia Perennis, 2003).

O'Dea, Kerin. "Marked Improvement in

Carbohydrate and Lipid Metabolism in Diabetic Australian Aborigines After Temporary Reversion to Traditional Life-style." *Diabetes.* 33 (1984): 596–603. This is the research referred to at the beginning of Part II. It is further elaborated on in:

————. "The Therapeutic and Preventive Potential of the Hunter-Gatherer Life-style: Insights from Australian Aborigines." From *Western Diseases.* Edited by N. J. Temple and D. P. Burkitt (Totowa, NJ: Humana Press, 1994).

Perry, George H., et al. "Diet and the Evolution of Human Amylase Gene Copy Number Variation." *Nature Genetics.* doi:10.1038/ng2123 (September 9, 2007).

Price, Weston A. *Nutrition and Physical Degeneration,* 7th edition (LaMesa: Price-Pottenger Nutrition Foundation, Inc., 2006).

Renner, Martin. "Modern Civilization, Nutritional Dark Age: Weston A. Price's Ecological Critique of the Industrial Food System" (UC Santa Cruz master's thesis, 2005).

Schmid, Ronald F. *Traditional Foods Are Your Best Medicine: Improving Health and Longevity with Native Nutrition* (Rochester, NY: Healing Arts Press, 1987).

Taubes, Gary. *Good Calories, Bad Calories* (New York: Knopf, 2007). See Chapter 5, "The Diseases of Civilization."

Western Diseases. Edited by Norman J. Temple and Denis P. Burkitt (Totowa, NJ: Humana Press Inc., 1994).

On the industrialization of agriculture and the links between soil and health:

Asami, Danny K., et al. "Comparison of the Total Phenolic and Ascorbic Acid Content of Freeze-Dried and Air-Dried Marion-berry, Strawberry, and Corn Using Conventional, Organic, and Sustainable Agricultural Practices." *Journal of Agricultural and Food Chemistry.* 51 (2003): 1237–41.

Benbrook, Charles M. "Elevating Antioxidant Levels in Food Through Organic Farming and Food Processing: An Organic Center State of Science Review" (Foster, RI: Organic Center, 2005).

Berry, Wendell. *The Unsettling of America: Culture and Agriculture* (San Francisco: Sierra Club Books, 1977).

Brandt, Kirsten, and Jens Peter Mølgaard. "Organic Agriculture: Does It Enhance or Reduce the Nutritional Value of Plant Foods?" *Journal of the Science of Food and*

Agriculture. 81.9 (2001): 924–31.

Carbonaro, Marina, and Maria Mattera. "Polyphenoloxidase Activity and Polyphenol Levels in Organically and Conventionally Grown Peaches." *Food Chemistry.* 72 (2001): 419–24.

Davis, Donald R., et al. "Changes in USDA Food Composition Data for 43 Garden Crops, 1950 to 1999." *Journal of the American College of Nutrition.* 23.6 (2004): 669–82.

———. "Trade-Offs in Agriculture and Nutrition." *Food Technology.* 59.3 (2005).

Fox, Jennifer E., et al. "Pesticides Reduce Symbiotic Efficiency of Nitrogen-Fixing Rhizobia and Host Plants." *Proceedings of the National Academy of Sciences.* 104.24 (2007).

Garvin, David F., Ross M. Welch, and John W. Finley. "Historical Shifts in the Seed Mineral Micronutrient Concentration of US Hard Red Winter Wheat Germplasm." *Journal of the Science of Food and Agriculture.* 86 (2006): 2213–20.

Halweil, Brian. "Still No Free Lunch: Nutrient Content of U.S. Food Supply Suffers at Hands of High Yields" (Foster, RI: Organic Center, 2007). An excellent survey of the literature.

Harvey, Graham. *The Forgiveness of Nature:*

The Story of Grass (London: Jonathan Cape/Random House, 2001).

Howard, Sir Albert. *An Agricultural Testament* (New York: Oxford University Press, 1943).

———. *The Soil and Health* (Lexington, KY: The University of Kentucky Press, 2006).

Manning, Richard. *Against the Grain* (New York: North Point Press, 2004).

Mayer, Anne-Marie. "Historical Changes in the Mineral Content of Fruits and Vegetables." *British Food Journal.* 99.6 (1997): 207–11.

Mitchell, Alyson E., et al. "Ten-Year Comparison of the Influences of Organic and Conventional Crop Management Practices on the Content of Flavonoids in Tomatoes." *Journal of Food and Agricultural Chemistry* (published online June 23, 2007).

Murphy, K., et al. "Relationship Between Yield and Mineral Nutrient Content in Historical and Modern Spring Wheat Cultivars." *Plant Genetic Resources* (in press).

Pollan, Michael. *The Botany of Desire: A Plant's-Eye View of the World* (New York: Random House, 2001).

———. *The Omnivore's Dilemma: A Natural History of Four Meals* (New York: Penguin

Press, 2006).

Ryan, M.H., et al. "Grain Mineral Concentrations and Yield of Wheat Grown Under Organic and Conventional Management." *Journal of the Science of Food and Agriculture.* 84 (2004): 207–16.

Schmid, Ronald. *The Untold Story of Milk* (Washington, D.C.: New Trends Publishing Inc., 2007).

Voisin, André. *Soil, Grass and Cancer* (Austin: Acres U.S.A., Publishers, 1999).

White, P.J., and M. R. Broadley. "Historical Variation in the Mineral Composition of Edible Horticultural Products." *Journal of Horticultural Science & Biotechnology.* 80.6 (2005): 660–67.

For statistical information on twentieth-century changes in the American food supply and diet:

U.N. Food and Agriculture Organization (FAO). FAOSTAT Statistical Database: "Agriculture/Production/Core Production Data." Accessed online at http://faostat.fao.org.

USDA Economic Research Service. "Major Trends in U.S. Food Supply, 1909–99." *FoodReview.* 23.1 (2000).

———. "U.S. Food Supply Providing More Food and Calories." *FoodReview.* 22.3 (1999).

———. "U.S. per Capita Food Supply Trends: More Calories, Refined Carbohydrates, and Fats." *FoodReview.* 25.3 (2002).

On the health implications of various dietary patterns (as opposed to individual nutrients):

Ames, Bruce N. "Increasing Longevity by Tuning Up Metabolism." *European Molecular Biology Organization.* 6 (2005): S20–S24. More of Ames' research on micronutrient deficiencies is available at his Web site: www.bruceames.org.

———. "Low Micronutrient Intake May Accelerate the Degenerative Diseases of Aging Through Allocation of Scarce Micronutrients by Triage." *Proceedings of the National Academy of Sciences.* 103.47 (2006): 17589–94.

Appel, Lawrence J. "A Clinical Trial of the Effects of Dietary Patterns on Blood Pressure." *New England Journal of Medicine.* 336.16 (1997): 1117–24.

de Lorgeril, Michel. "Mediterranean Diet,

Traditional Risk Factors, and the Rate of Cardiovascular Complications After Myocardial Infarction: Final Report of the Lyon Diet Heart Study." *Journal of the American Heart Association.* 99 (1999): 779–85.

Jacobs, David R., et al. "Nutrients, Foods, and Dietary Patterns as Exposures in Research: A Framework for Food Synergy." *American Journal of Clinical Nutrition.* 78 suppl (2003): 508S–13S. This is the study on whole grains discussed in the section.

Liu, Simin, et al. "Fruit and Vegetable Intake and Risk of Cardiovascular Disease: The Women's Health Study." *American Journal of Clinical Nutrition.* 72 (2000): 922–28.

Planck, Nina. *Real Food: What to Eat and Why* (New York: Bloomsbury, 2006).

Weil, Andrew. *Healthy Aging: A Lifelong Guide to Your Physical and Spiritual Well-Being* (New York: Knopf, 2005).

On the rise of modern processed foods:

Drummond, J.C. *The Englishman's Food: A History of Five Centuries of English Diet* (Oxford: Alden Press, 1939).

Levenstein, Harvey. *Paradox of Plenty: A Social History of Eating in Modern America* (Berkeley: University of California Press, 2003).

———. *Revolution at the Table: The Transformation of the American Diet* (Berkeley: University of California Press, 2003).

Perren, Richard. "Structural Change and Market Growth in the Food Industry: Flour Milling in Britain, Europe, and America, 1850–1914." *Economic History Review.* 43.3 (1990): 420–37.

Shapiro, Laura. *Perfection Salad: Women and Cooking at the Turn of the Century* (New York: Random House, 2001).

———. *Something from the Oven: Reinventing Dinner in 1950s America* (New York: Penguin, 2005).

Tannahill, Reay. *Food in History* (New York: Stein and Day, 1973).

Tisdale, Sally. *The Best Thing I Ever Tasted: The Secret of Food* (New York: Riverhead, 2001).

On omega-3 and omega-6 fatty acids:

Allport, Susan. *The Queen of Fats: Why Omega-3s Were Removed from the Western Diet and What We Can Do to Replace Them*

(Berkeley: University of California Press, 2006). By far the best work of science journalism on the subject.

————. "The Skinny on Fat." *Gastronomica — The Journal of Food and Culture.* 3.1 (2003): 28–36.

Carlson, Susan E., and Martha Neuringer. "Polyunsaturated Fatty Acid and Neurodevelopment: A Summary and Critical Analysis of the Literature." *Lipids.* 34.2 (1999): 171–78.

Hibbeln, J.R., et al. "Dietary Polyunsaturated Fatty Acids and Depression: When Cholesterol Doesn't Satisfy." *American Journal of Clinical Nutrition.* 62 (1995): 1–9.

————, et al. "Healthy Intakes of n-3 and n-6 Fatty Acids: Estimations Considering Worldwide Diversity." *American Journal of Clinical Nutrition.* 83 (2006).

————, et al. "Increasing Homicide Rates and Linoleic Acid Consumption Among Five Western Countries, 1961–2000." *Lipids.* 39.12 (2004).

Holman, Ralph T. "The Slow Discovery of the Importance of Omega-3 Fatty Acids in Human Health." Presented as part of a symposium, "Evolution of Ideas About the Nutritional Value of Dietary Fat," at the Experimental Biology 97 meeting, April

9, 1997. The proceedings were published by the American Society for Nutritional Sciences in 1998.

Kris-Etherton, P.M., et al. "Polyunsaturated Fatty Acids in the Food Chain in the United States." *American Journal of Clinical Nutrition.* 71 (2000): 179S–88S.

Mozaffarian, Dariush, and Eric B. Rimm. "Fish Intake, Contaminants, and Human Health: Evaluating the Risks and the Benefits." *Journal of the American Medical Association.* 296.15 (2006): 1885–99.

Nesheim, Malden C., et al. "Seafood Choices: Balancing Benefits and Risks" (Washington D.C.: National Academies Press, 2006).

Pischon, Tobias, et al. "Habitual Dietary Intake of n-3 and n-6 Fatty Acids in Relation to Inflammatory Markers Among US Men and Women." *Circulation.* 108 (2003): 155–60.

Simopoulos, Artemis P., and Jo Robinson. *The Omega Diet: The Lifesaving Nutritional Program Based on the Diet of the Island of Crete* (New York: HarperCollins, 1998).

Uauy, Ricardo, et al. "Essential Fatty Acids in Visual and Brain Development." *Lipids.* 36.9 (2001): 885–95.

On the rising incidence of type 2 diabetes and its impact:

Boyle, James P., et al. "Projection of Diabetes Burden Through 2050: Impact of Changing Demography and Disease Prevalence in the U.S." *Diabetes Care.* 24 (2001): 1936–40.

Gregg, Edward W., et al. "Trends in the Prevalence and Ratio of Diagnosed to Undiagnosed Diabetes According to Obesity Levels in the U.S." *Diabetes Care.* 27 (2004): 2806–12.

Haslam, David W., and W. Philip T. James. "Obesity." *The Lancet.* 336 (2005): 1197–1209.

Kleinfield, N.R. "Diabetes and Its Awful Toll Quietly Emerge as a Crisis." *The New York Times* (January 9, 2006).

———. "Living at an Epicenter of Diabetes, Defiance and Despair." *New York Times* (January 10, 2006).

Narayan, K. M. Venkat, et al. "Lifetime Risk for Diabetes Mellitus in the United States." *Journal of the American Medical Association.* 290.14 (2003): 1884–90.

O'Connor, Andrew S., and Jeffrey R. Schelling. "Diabetes and the Kidney." *American Journal of Kidney Diseases.* 46.4 (2005): 766–73.

Olshansky, S. Jay, et al. "A Potential Decline in Life Expectancy in the United States in the 21st Century." *New England Journal of Medicine.* 352.11 (2005): 1138–45.

Poinasamy, Darren. "Facing Up to the Diabetes Threat in the US." *Business Briefing: US Pharmacy Review.* (2004): 48–50.

Urbina, Ian. "In the Treatment of Diabetes, Success Often Does Not Pay." *New York Times* (January 11, 2006).

Wild, Sarah, et al. "Global Prevalence of Diabetes: Estimates for the Year 2000 and Projections for 2030." *Diabetes Care.* 27.5 (2004): 1047–53.

Part Three: Getting Over Nutritionism
1. Eat Food: On the benefits of whole foods and traditional diets:

Allport, Susan. *The Primal Feast: Food, Sex, Foraging, and Love* (Lincoln, NB: iUniverse Inc., 2000).

American Journal of Clinical Nutrition. Edited by Marion Nestle, et al. 61 suppl (1995): 1313–20. This special supplement edition looked at the benefits of the Mediterranean diet.

Appel, Lawrence J. "A Clinical Trial of the Effects of Dietary Patterns on Blood Pressure." *New England Journal of Medicine.* 336.16 (1997): 1117–24.

Brown, Melody J., et al. "Carotenoid Bioavailability Is Higher from Salads Ingested with Full-Fat Than with Fat-Reduced Salad Dressings as Measured with Electrochemical Detection." *American Journal of Clinical Nutrition.* 80 (2004): 396–403.

de Lorgeril, Michel. "Mediterranean Diet, Traditional Risk Factors, and the Rate of Cardiovascular Complications After Myocardial Infarction: Final Report of the Lyon Diet Heart Study." *Journal of the American Heart Association.* 99 (1999): 779–85.

Feenstra, Gail. "The Roles of Farmers' Markets in Fueling Local Economies." *Gastronomic Sciences.* 1 (2007).

Fielding, Jeanette M., and Kerin O' Dea, et al. "Increases in Plasma Lycopene Concentration After Consumption of Tomatoes Cooked with Olive Oil." *Asia Pacific Journal of Clinical Nutrition.* 14.2 (2005): 131–36.

Gussow, Joan Dye. "Why You Should Eat Food, and Other Nutritional Heresies." Speech, University of California, Davis, Plant & Environmental Sciences. November 7, 2003.

Hu, Frank B., et al. "Prospective Study of

Major Dietary Patterns and Risk of Coronary Heart Disease in Men." *American Journal of Clinical Nutrition.* 72 (2002): 912–21.

Johnston, Francis E. "Food and Biocultural Evolution: A Model for the Investigation of Modern Nutritional Problems." *Nutritional Anthropology* (Philadelphia: University of Pennsylvania, 1987).

Kouris-Blazos, Antigone, et al. "Are the Advantages of the Mediterranean Diet Transferable to Other Populations? A Cohort Study in Melbourne, Australia." *British Journal of Nutrition.* 82 (1999): 57–61.

Milburn, Michael P. "Indigenous Nutrition." *American Indian Quarterly.* 28.3 (2004): 411–34.

Nabhan, Gary Paul. *Why Some Like It Hot: Food, Genes, and Cultural Diversity* (Washington, D.C.: Island Press, 2004).

Nestle, Marion. *What to Eat* (New York: North Point Press, 2006).

Planck, Nina. *Real Food: What to Eat and Why* (New York: Bloomsbury, 2006).

Sherman, Paul W., and Jennifer Billing. "Darwinian Gastronomy: Why We Use Spices." *Bioscience.* 49.6 (1999): 453–63.

Simopoulos, Artemis P. "The Mediterranean Diets: What Is So Special About the Diet of Greece? The Scientific Evidence." *Journal of Nutrition*. (American Institute for Cancer Research 11th Annual Research Conference on Diet, Nutrition and Cancer, Washington, D.C., July 16–17, 2001): 3065S–73S.

————, and Jo Robinson. *The Omega Diet: The Lifesaving Nutritional Program Based on the Diet of the Island of Crete* (New York: HarperCollins, 1998).

Trichopoulou, A., and E. Vasilopoulou. "Mediterranean Diet and Longevity." *British Journal of Nutrition*. 84 suppl. 2 (2000): S205–S9.

Unlu, Nuray Z., et al. "Carotenoid Absorption from Salad and Salsa by Humans Is Enhanced by the Addition of Avocado or Avocado Oil." *Journal of Nutrition*. 135 (2005): 431–36.

van het Hof, Karin H., et al. "Dietary Factors That Affect the Bioavailability of Carotenoids." *Journal of Nutrition*. 130 (2000): 503–6.

Willett, Walter C. "Diet and Health: What Should We Eat?" *Science*. 264.5158 (1994): 532–37.

On processed foods and health claims:

Barrionuevo, Alexei. "Globalization in Every Loaf." *New York Times* (June 16, 2007). A good account of Sara Lee's whole-grain white bread. See also: www.thejoyofeating .com/.

Erdman, John W., et al. "Not All Soy Products Are Created Equal: Caution Needed in Interpretation of Research Results" (Fifth International Symposium on the Role of Soy in Preventing and Treating Chronic Disease, American Society for Nutrition Sciences, 2004).

Holvoet, Paul, et al. "Circulating Oxidized LDL Is a Useful Marker for Identifying Patients with Coronary Artery Disease." *Arteriosclerosis, Thrombosis, and Vascular Biology.* 21 (2001): 844–48.

Hur, S.J., et al. "Formation of Cholesterol Oxidation Products (COPs) in animal products." *Food Control.* 18 (2007): 939–47.

Lesser, L.I., D.S. Ludwig, et al. "Relationship Between Funding Source and Conclusion Among Nutrition-Related Scientific Articles." *Public Library of Science.* 4.1, e5 doi:10.1371/journal.pmed. 0040005 (2007).

Martin, Andrew. "Makers of Sodas Try a

New Pitch: They're Healthy." *New York Times* (March 7, 2007).

Messina, Mark J. "Legumes and Soybeans: Overview of Their Nutritional Profiles and Health Effects." *American Journal of Clinical Nutrition.* 70 (1999): 439S–50S.

Pie, Jae Eun, et al. "Evaluation of Oxidative Degradation of Cholesterol in Food and Food Ingredients: Identification and Quantification of Cholesterol Oxides." *Journal of Agriculture and Food Chemistry.* 38 (1990): 973–79.

Ravn, Karen. "Corn Oil's 'Qualified Health Claim' Raises Eyebrows." *Los Angeles Times* (April 16, 2007).

Staprans, Ilona, et al. "The Role of Dietary Oxidized Cholesterol and Oxidized Fatty Acids in the Development of Atherosclerosis." *Molecular Nutrition and Food Research.* 49 (2005): 1075–82.

Tenbergen, Klaus. "Dough and Bread Conditioners." *Food Product Design — Culinary Connection.* Accessed online August 1, 2007 at http://www.foodproductdesign .com/archive/1999/1199cc.html.

U.S. FDA. Qualified Health Claims: Letter of Enforcement Discretion — Corn Oil and Oil-Containing Products and a Reduced Risk of Heart Disease (Docket No.

2006P-0243). Accessed online July 21, 2007 at http://www.cfsan.fda.gov/~dms/qhccorno.html.

U.S. FDA. Letter responding to health claim petition dated August 28, 2003: Monounsaturated Fatty Acids from Olive Oil and Coronary Heart Disease (Docket No. 2003Q-0559). Accessed online July 21, 2007 at http://www.cfsan.fda.gov/~dms/qhcolive.html.

Warner, Melanie. "Science's Quest to Banish Fat in Tasty Ways." *New York Times* (August 11, 2005).

2. Mostly Plants: On plant-based diets and meat eating:

Appel, Lawrence J. "A Clinical Trial of the Effects of Dietary Patterns on Blood Pressure." *New England Journal of Medicine.* 336.16 (1997): 1117–24.

Campbell, T. Colin, and Thomas M. Campbell II. *The China Study* (Dallas: BenBella Books, Inc., 2006).

Cho, Eunyoung, Sc.D., et al. "Red Meat Intake and Risk of Breast Cancer Among Postmenopausal Women." *Archives of Internal Medicine.* 166 (2006): 2253–59.

Gardner, Christopher D. "The Effect of a

Plant-Based Diet on Plasma Lipids in Hypercholesterolemic Adults." *Annals of Internal Medicine.* 142 (2005): 725–33.

Greene, Kelly. "Aging Well: How to Eat Meat and Still Feel as Healthy as a Vegetarian." *Wall Street Journal* (October 21, 2006).

Heber, David. *What Color Is Your Diet?* (New York: ReganBooks, 2001). Excellent discussion of antioxidants and the benefits of a plant-based diet.

Hu, Frank B., et al. "Frequent Nut Consumption and Risk of Coronary Heart Disease in Women: Prospective Cohort Study." *British Medical Journal.* 317 (1998): 1341–45.

———. "Plant-Based Foods and Prevention of Cardiovascular Disease: An Overview. *American Journal of Clinical Nutrition.* 78 suppl (2003): 544S–51S.

Jacobs, David R., and Lyn M. Steffen. "Nutrients, Foods, and Dietary Patterns as Exposures in Research: A Framework for Food Synergy." *American Journal of Clinical Nutrition.* 78.3 (2003): 508S–13S.

Jacobson, Michael F., and the staff of the Center for Science in the Public Interest. *Six Arguments for a Greener Diet: How a More Plant-Based Diet Could Save Your Health and the Environment* (Washington,

D.C.: Center for Science in the Public Interest, 2006).

Key, Timothy J. A., et al. "Dietary Habits and Mortality in 11,000 Vegetarians and Health Conscious People: Results of a 17-Year Follow-up." *British Medical Journal.* 313 (1996): 775–79.

Key, Timothy J., et al. "Health Effects of Vegetarian and Vegan Diets." *Proceedings of the Nutrition Society.* 65 (2006): 35–41.

Leitzmann, Claus. "Nutrition Ecology: The Contribution of Vegetarian Diets." *American Journal of Clinical Nutrition.* 78 suppl (2003): 657S–59S.

Newby, P.K., et al. "Risk of Overweight and Obesity Among Semivegetarian, Lactovegetarian, and Vegan Women." *American Journal of Clinical Nutrition.* 81 (2005): 1267–74.

Steinfeld, Henning, et al. *Livestock's Long Shadow: Environmental Issues and Options.* A report published by the Food and Agriculture Organization of the United Nations (Rome: FAO, 2006). Available online at http://www.virtualcentre.org/en/library/keypub/longshad/A0701E00.htm.

Willett, Walter C. "Diet and Health: What Should We Eat?" *Science.* 264.5158

(1994): 532–37.

3. Not Too Much: On Eating habits, food culture, and health:

Berry, Wendell. "The Pleasures of Eating," in *What Are People For?* (New York: North Point Press, 1990).

———. "The Reactor and the Garden," in *The Gift of Good Land* (San Francisco: North Point Press, 1981). On the political significance of gardening.

Brillat-Savarin, Jean-Anthelme. *The Physiology of Taste.* Translated by Anne Drayton (London: Penguin, 1994).

Cutler, David M., et al. "Why Have Americans Become More Obese?" *Journal of Economic Perspectives.* 17.3 (2003): 93–118.

Geier, Andrew B., and Paul Rozin, et al. "Unit Bias: A New Heuristic That Helps Explain the Effect of Portion Size on Food Intake." *Psychological Science.* 17.6 (2006): 521–25.

Hartman, Harvey, and Jarrett Paschel. "Understanding Obesity: Practical Suggestions for the Obesity Crisis" (Bellevue, WA: The Hartman Group, Inc., 2006).

Katz, Sandor Ellix. *The Revolution Will Not*

320

Be Microwaved (White River Junction, VT: Chelsea Green, 2007).

Montanari, Massimo. *Food Is Culture* (New York: Columbia University Press, 2006).

Petrini, Carlo. *Slow Food Nation* (New York: Rizzoli Ex Libris, 2007). For more on the Slow Food movement, see its Web site: www.Slowfood.com.

———. "Terra Madre Opening Speech." Turin, Italy. October 20, 2004.

Pollan, Michael. "Cruising on the Ark of Taste." *Mother Jones* (May, 2003).

Rozin, Paul, et al. "The Ecology of Eating: Smaller Portion Sizes in France Than in the United States Help Explain the French Paradox." *Psychological Science*. 14.5 (2003): 450–54.

———, et al. "Food and Life, Pleasure and Worry, Among American College Students: Gender Differences and Regional Similarities." *Journal of Personality and Social Psychology*. 85.1 (2003): 132–41.

Wansink, Brian. *Mindless Eating: Why We Eat More Than We Think* (New York: Bantam Books, 2006).

On calorie restriction:

Civitarese, Anthony E. "Calorie Restriction

Increases Muscle Mitochondrial Biogenesis in Healthy Humans." *Public Library of Science.* 4.3 (2007): 0485–94.

"Eat Your Cake and Have It" (New York: Nature Publishing Group, 2006).

Fontana, Luigi. "Excessive Adiposity, Calorie Restriction, and Aging." *Journal of the American Medical Association.* 295.13 (2006): 1577–78.

Heilbronn, Leonie K., et al. "Effect of 6-Month Calorie Restriction on Biomarkers of Longevity, Metabolic Adaptation, and Oxidative Stress in Overweight Individuals." *Journal of the American Medical Association.* 295.13 (2006): 1539–48.

Meyer, Timothy E., et al. "Long-Term Caloric Restriction Ameliorates the Decline in Diastolic Function in Humans." *Journal of the American College of Cardiology.* 47.2 (2006): 398–402.

Seligman, Katherine. "Iron Will." *San Francisco Chronicle* (September 2, 2007).

On drinking and the French paradox:

Criqui, M.H., and Brenda L. Ringel. "Does Diet or Alcohol Explain the French Paradox?" *The Lancet.* 344 (1994): 8939–40.

Drewnowski, Adam, et al. "Diet Quality and

Dietary Diversity in France: Implications for the French Paradox." *Journal of the American Dietetic Association.* 96.7 (1996): 663–69.

Ferrieres, Jean. "The French Paradox: Lessons for Other Countries." *Heart.* 90 (2004): 107–11.

Fuchs, Flavio D. "Vascular Effects of Alcoholic Beverages: Is It Only Alcohol That Matters?" *Hypertension.* 45 (2005): 851–52.

Mukamal, Kenneth J., et al. "Roles of Drinking Pattern and Type of Alcohol Consumed in Coronary Heart Disease in Men." *New England Journal of Medicine.* 348.2 (2003): 109–18.

Opie, Lionel H., and Sandrine Lecour. "The Red Wine Hypothesis: From Concepts to Protective Signalling Molecules." *European Heart Journal.* 28 (2007): 1683–93.

Renaud, S., and M. de Lorgeril. "Wine, Alcohol, Platelets, and the French Paradox for Coronary Heart Disease." *The Lancet.* 339.8808 (1992): 1523–26.

Rimm, E. "Commentary: Alcohol and Coronary Heart Disease — Laying the Foundation for Future Work." *International Journal of Epidemiology.* 30 (2001): 738–39.

Volatier, Jean-Luc, and Philippe Verger.

"Recent National French Food and Nutrient Intake Data." *British Journal of Nutrition.* 81.S2 (1999): 57–59.

Zuger, Abigail. "The Case for Drinking (All Together Now: In Moderation!)." *New York Times* (December 31, 2002).

———. "How a Tonic Keeps the Parts Well Oiled." *New York Times* (December 31, 2002).

RESOURCES

A selection of resources for finding real food and eating locally:

Print

Damrosch, Barbara. *The Garden Primer: Second Edition* (New York: Workman, 2008).

Edible Communities. A network of excellent local magazines on local food. For more information: www.ediblecommunities.com.

Gussow, Joan Dye. *This Organic Life: Confessions of a Suburban Homesteader* (White River Junction, VT: Chelsea Green, 2001).

Jeavons, John. *How to Grow More Vegetables* (Berkeley: Ten Speed Press, 2006).

Kingsolver, Barbara, et al. *Animal, Vegetable, Miracle: A Year of Food Life* (New York: HarperCollins, 2007).

McKibben, Bill. *Deep Economy: The Wealth of Communities and the Durable Future*

(New York: Henry Holt and Company, LLC, 2007).

Madison, Deborah. *Local Flavors: Cooking and Eating from America's Farmer's Markets* (New York: Broadway Books, 2002).

Nabhan, Gary Paul. *Coming Home to Eat: The Pleasures and Politics of Local Foods* (New York: W. W. Norton, 2002).

Peterson, John, and Angelic Organics. *Farmer John's Cookbook: The Real Dirt on Vegetables* (Salt Lake City: Gibbs Smith, Publisher, 2006).

Salatin, Joel. *Holy Cows and Hog Heaven: The Food Buyer's Guide to Farm-Fresh Food* (Swoope, VA: Polyface, 2006).

Web

Center for Informed Food Choices (www.informedeating.org) advocates for a diet based on whole, unprocessed, local, organically grown plant foods; their Web site contains a useful FAQ page about food politics and eating well in addition to an archive of relevant articles.

Eat Local Challenge (www.eatlocal challenge.com) offers resources and encouragement for people trying to eat locally.

Eat Well (www.eatwellguide.com) is an online directory of sustainably raised meat, poultry, dairy, and eggs. Enter your zip code to find healthful, humane, and ecofriendly products from farms, stores, and restaurants in your area.

Eat Wild (www.eatwild.com) lists local suppliers for grass-fed meat and dairy products.

Food Routes (www.foodroutes.org) is a national nonprofit dedicated to "reintroducing Americans to their food — the seeds it grows from, the farmers who produce it, and the routes that carry it from the fields to our tables."

Local Harvest (www.localharvest.com) helps you connect with local farmers, CSAs, and farmers' markets.

Weston A. Price Foundation (www .westonaprice.org) is an archive of information on the sorts of traditional whole-food diets advocated by Weston A. Price. Local chapters are good resources on where to find some of the best pastured animal foods.

ABOUT THE AUTHOR

Michael Pollan is the author of four previous books, including *The Omnivore's Dilemma* and *The Botany of Desire,* both *New York Times* bestsellers. A longtime contributor to *The New York Times Magazine,* he is also the Knight Professor of Journalism at Berkeley. To read more of his work, go to www.michaelpollan.com

The employees of Thorndike Press hope you have enjoyed this Large Print book. All our Thorndike and Wheeler Large Print titles are designed for easy reading, and all our books are made to last. Other Thorndike Press Large Print books are available at your library, through selected bookstores, or directly from us.

For information about titles, please call:
  (800) 223-1244

or visit our Web site at:
  http://gale.cengage.com/thorndike

To share your comments, please write:
  Publisher
  Thorndike Press
  295 Kennedy Memorial Drive
  Waterville, ME 04901